The Vitamin Cure for Eye Disease

Robert G. Smith, Ph.D.
Andrew W. Saul, Ph.D., Series Editor

16
EasyRead Large

RHYW

Copyright Page from the Original Book

The information contained in this book is based upon the research and personal and professional experiences of the authors. It is not intended as a substitute for consulting with your physician or other healthcare provider. Any attempt to diagnose and treat an illness should be done under the direction of a healthcare professional.

The publisher does not advocate the use of any particular healthcare protocol but believes the information in this book should be available to the public. The publisher and authors are not responsible for any adverse effects or consequences resulting from the use of the suggestions, preparations, or procedures discussed in this book. Should the reader have any questions concerning the appropriateness of any procedures or preparation mentioned, the authors and the publisher strongly suggest consulting a professional healthcare advisor.

Basic Health Publications, Inc.
28812 Top of the World Drive
Laguna Beach, CA 92651
949–715–7327 • www.basichealthpub.com

Library of Congress Cataloging-in-Publication Data

Smith, Robert G.
The vitamin cure for eye disease / Robert G. Smith.
p. cm.
Includes bibliographical references and index.
ISBN 978-1-59120-292-9
1. Eye—Diseases—Alternative treatment—Popular works. 2. Vitamin therapy—Popular works. 3. Eye—Diseases—Diet therapy—Popular works.
I. Title.
RE51.S65 2012
617.7'06—dc23

2012014007

Editor: Diana Drew
Typesetting/Book design: Gary A. Rosenberg
Cover design: Mike Stromberg

Printed in the United States of America

10 9 8 7 6 5 4 3 2 1

TABLE OF CONTENTS

ACKNOWLEDGMENTS

This book is based on my paper "Nutrition and eye disease" published in the *Journal of Orthomolecular Medicine,* Third Quarter, 2010. I thank *JOM* Managing Editor Steve Carter for permission to use the material in the paper. I thank Basic Health's *Vitamin Cure* series editor Andrew W. Saul for encouragement, and publisher Norman R. Goldfind for his foresight in developing the Basic Health series of books. I thank Thomas E. Levy, M.D., for his generous and helpful words in the foreword. I thank my parents for getting me interested in science, health, and eating right; Joe Cadbury for showing me nature and how to study it; Peter Sterling for our long-term collaboration in retinal circuitry; my colleagues in retinal circuitry for their impassioned pursuit of the truth; and Michael Chaitin for showing me and many others how to get organized.

FOREWORD

Vision is something we tend to take for granted until it begins to deteriorate. It is at that point that our quality of vision becomes profoundly important. After all, there are few people who would consider the loss of any sense or body part more important than vision.

But too often we don't behave as if it really *is* that important, as long as we have no ongoing problems with it. Unlike with, say, heart disease, few people respect their good vision enough to practice preventive medicine in order to preserve it. Yet most people would be much more apprehensive over completely losing their vision in later life than they would fear the increasing chances of having a fatal heart attack. Nevertheless, many middle-aged individuals these days are going to great lengths with exercise, diet, supplementation, and prescription drugs to forestall the onset of heart disease, while doing virtually nothing specific to help preserve their good vision.

In this book, Dr. Smith describes how a great variety of eye diseases take hold and progress over time. His writing is clear and concise, and he is very effective in teaching a subject that he obviously knows very well. Good teachers are like that. Far more teachers, unfortunately, may still know their subject well, yet they just do not have the ability to relate it to a student in both simple words and clear concepts. This book taught me, a physician, a great deal about a subject that I should have known better, but did not. I suppose this is why so many specialties and subspecialties exist in medicine. There really isn't time to know everything of importance. Or maybe, as a cardiologist, that's just my excuse!

So why is a cardiologist writing the foreword to an eye diseases book? In my own research, it has become increasingly apparent to me over time that all diseases—every single one—start when there is enough excess oxidative stress in the wrong place at the wrong time. It is the maintenance of that excess oxidative stress that permits diseases to evolve and worsen the longer it is present. No exceptions. In *The Vitamin Cure for Eye Disease,* Dr. Smith presents the scientific case for what I always suspected, but had never taken the time to learn. Specifically, he shows how most, if not all, significant eye diseases both start and progress because of excess oxidative stress in a given part of the eye. Furthermore, he makes a strong case that bolstering the antioxidant capacity of the eye is probably the single best way to not only forestall the onset of eye disease, but also to slow or prevent its progression if the disease process has already started.

This book makes a solid contribution to the growing evidence that excess oxidative stress is our body's main enemy, and that maintaining high levels of the most important antioxidants, led by vitamin C, is the single most important thing we can do to not only live long and well, but to have excellent vision during that life. Dr. Smith should be commended for this excellent work.

Thomas E. Levy, M.D., J.D.

CHAPTER 1

HOW VITAMINS CAN HELP OUR HEALTH: AN INTRODUCTION

In his book, *Doctor Yourself,* nutritionist and author Andrew W. Saul describes the recovery of one of his clients from a progressive eye disease.[1] The woman, in her thirties, had been losing her peripheral vision. She had been told by her eye doctor that further loss was inevitable but that nothing could be done about it. She was desperate. After considering her case history and her personal eating habits, Dr. Saul advised her to eat raw foods, especially sprouts, and although she didn't like the idea, she resolved to try it. Saul explained how she could purchase inexpensive seeds and sprout them, eating several jars of different kinds of juicy, crunchy sprouts each day. Although the woman had misgivings and many questions, she gradually learned new eating habits and maintained the raw food diet over the weeks and months that followed. At first she hated eating raw sprouts, but soon learned to eat generous amounts of them prepared in different ways according to her taste. And of course she ate other nutritious food too, like yogurt and chicken, as well as a few selected vitamin and mineral supplements. Eventually she worked up to eating several quarts of sprouts each day along with whatever else made them inviting and tasty. According to her ophthalmologist, her eyesight didn't get any worse over the next few months. Then, gradually, a miracle seemed to happen—over a period of many months on this regimen, her eyesight progressively returned, finally becoming almost normal. Without any other treatment, she had recovered.

This book is about how to treat eye disease and prevent its occurrence through good nutrition. Many eye conditions and diseases are considered to be progressive, meaning that once their typical symptoms are identified, they usually get worse. Although drug treatments exist for these eye diseases, generally the drugs do not cure, and typically they can only slow the progression. The reason is that many eye diseases are "age-related," meaning that their symptoms threaten sight late in life, typically after age fifty to sixty.[2] On first thought this might seem to imply these diseases are caused by the aging process. However, age related eye diseases have several causes. Some of them are not inevitable but can be prevented. In many eye diseases, normal wear and tear to the eye over a lifetime damages it beyond repair. Our eyes are at a heavy risk for damage because they sit at the periphery of the body and so are exposed to environmental toxins. Moreover, the eye is prone to disease because it is exposed to bright sunlight, which is known to damage biological molecules. Many age-related eye diseases are accelerated by genetic abnormalities that impair the eye's ability to repair itself. Finally, the neural tissue at the back of the eye has a relatively high metabolism and a high content of polyunsaturated fatty acids. This puts it at extra risk for disease. All of these factors can be ameliorated through nutrition.

ORTHOMOLECULAR MEDICINE

Proper nutrition can prevent disease and help you stay healthy. Orthomolecular medicine is the practice of providing essential nutrients in sufficient quantity to prevent and cure illness. When the body is provided with optimal nutrition, it can metabolize food more efficiently to prevent the effects of harmful environmental toxins and disease. With a sufficient quantity of nutrients, such as vitamins and essential macro- and micro-minerals, either in food or supplements, it can stay healthier and prevent, to a large extent, age-related diseases such as cataracts, macular degeneration, and glaucoma. The reason is that vitamins and minerals, when taken along with a nutritious diet, help the body's maintenance and repair machinery keep its tissues healthier.[3] One way they do this is by removing the free radicals in the body's tissues that cause damage. Using natural molecules that the body needs for the normal processes of life, and taking them in sufficient quantities, orthomolecular medicine can prevent the damage caused by nutrient deficiencies and can help the body recover. Antioxidant vitamins C and E, taken over a person's lifetime in a sufficient quantity with other nutrients such as zinc, can prevent much age-related disease, especially in the eye.

In the popular literature, many authors advocate one or another particularly healthy diet, as in the example above using raw sprouts, or give simple but strict rules to follow: no refined foods such as sugar, flour, or oils, and no red or white meat. Several popular vegetarian diets have been proven to give excellent recovery from age-related vascular disease.[4] Other authors suggest that a normal balanced diet, with a variety of different types of foods, but without much refined food or meat, is all one needs to be healthy.[5] Some have further suggested that to discuss the benefits of specific nutrients is a symptom of our dependence on giant food corporations that vie to sell us refined food. After all, there are profits to be made in removing nutrients during the refining process and then adding them back again to provide health! Thus, some would have us believe that because a varied diet of natural foods is enough to keep us healthy, we don't need to, nor should we, categorize our food into separate nutrients.

Indeed, the body needs a variety of nutrients. A typical vegetable food such as a sprouted bean or leaf of kale contains a complex mixture of chemicals. They are so complex that their role in the body is difficult to determine. Very likely, some essential nutrients are still unidentified.[6] And from the evidence, eating lots of fruits, vegetables, whole grains, and other natural foods over a lifetime can help keep you healthy. But we also know that when food is digested by acid in the stomach and absorbed by the intestines, it is reduced to molecules. These comprise nutrients, some of which are vitamins and minerals necessary for our health. Some authors have written that tracking the separate nutrients is unnecessary because all we need is good food, but this seems to beg the question: which nutrients do we need, what combinations of them are most effective, and how can they prevent disease?[7] In this book we will explore the current knowledge about essential nutrients and how they can prevent eye diseases, so you can learn what nutrients are most likely to help.

The term *orthomolecular medicine* was coined by Linus Pauling, to mean the use of the "right" nutrients required by the body, in the correct amount and proportion to maintain health.[8] Pauling was the most famous chemist of the twentieth century, and one of the most important. In his 1986 book *How to Live Longer and Feel Better,* he described the scientific basis of orthomolecular medicine. His ideas were based on the work of many others, including several pioneers who discovered the benefits of high levels of nutrient supplements.[9] Pauling also based his view of orthomolecular medicine on his own voluminous knowledge of chemistry and healing from nutrition. He put forth the idea that we all have a requirement for nutrients, whether they are obtained from food or as supplements.

Pauling's insight into the levels of nutrients required by the body came from his knowledge that many nutrients are not used directly for energy, but are required as cofactors for enzymes that drive the reactions in the body's biochemical metabolic pathways. An excess of the vitamin cofactors assures that these reactions take place quickly and completely. This might seem counterintuitive, because one might imagine that an excess of nutrients would not be helpful to the body. For example, common sense tells us that eating too much food is not helpful to the body, because one would tend to put on excess weight, which is a risk factor for many diseases. However, the vitamin cofactors are necessary for supervising the generation of energy and the construction and maintenance of new cells and muscles. Thus, the levels of essential nutrients available to the body regulate, to a large extent, its ability to build and maintain itself.

To correctly perform its biochemical functions, the body requires adequate amounts of each essential nutrient. However, the exact amount of each nutrient required cannot be precisely defined as a single number because it differs widely among different individuals.[10] For "normal" people, the need for essential nutrients can vary up to eightyfold.[11] Yet, for most of these nutrients, having an excess of the enzymes, cofactors, and reactants for biochemical reactions is not harmful in any way. In fact, an excess can help the reaction take place faster and more robustly. For many biochemical pathways, a deficiency of any essential nutrient creates a "biochemical bottleneck." That is, when a deficiency of a nutrient limits one reaction in a biochemical pathway, it will likely also limit the rate of the entire pathway. A plentiful amount of the nutrient can keep the biochemical reactions flowing smoothly. For example, the B vitamins are required for the basic metabolic processes of the body such as maintaining, repairing, and growing. Under stressful conditions, these metabolic pathways are even more crucial. Thus, when taken at high levels known to be safe, the B vitamins are helpful to all tissues of the body.[12] Another example is the important nutrient magnesium, which is required for dozens of specific reactions. Its deficiency commonly causes a wide variety of symptoms.[13] So, by taking additional amounts of the nutrients we need the most, we allow our body to utilize our food more completely, to maintain itself and grow optimally, and to fight and prevent disease.

My Interest in Orthomolecular Medicine

My interest in nutrition began with my experiences as a young child. My early education about nutrition came from one of my teachers in grade school, who had an interest in health and nature. Throughout grade school, I always looked forward to “Nature” class, taught by Joe Cadbury, a man with an encyclopedic knowledge of nature and an avid birder. He explained the natural world to my class, encouraging us to ask questions that we would all try to answer together. We learned about dinosaurs, natural selection, and how different species evolved. He read the latest research articles and offered us selected stories about the latest studies of how animals live. He taught us about birds, their songs, what they ate, and where they build their nests to raise their young. He explained that some birds migrated to Central and South America during the winter to avoid the cold, but others survived in North America through the winter because they could find adequate nutrition. We learned about the senses, how we see and hear, how robins find worms (good eyesight), and how birds might sense magnetic fields when migrating.[14]

Mr. Cadbury took us to the local park along the Wissahickon Creek, showing us where trunks of dead chestnut trees lay after having been killed by the chestnut blight, still without much decay after sixty years. He showed us where live chestnuts still grew nearby from hardy root stock, and where bats, which have excellent night vision,[15] hid underneath loose bark of trees. We saw where ants and millipedes lived under logs. He took us to see tadpoles growing into frogs in a small pond. Mr. Cadbury was interested in how some species of birds survived very well in cities, and how others that needed wild habitats were becoming rare. As we got older, he invited us in the springtime to the woods at 7:00A.M. before school to listen for and identify the migrating birds. We learned the importance of careful listening and looking. He once quietly mentioned that an owl, a species with excellent night vision, lived in a hole in a tree behind the school, in the midst of the city! We were amazed and entertained by the fascinating stories about birds, animals, insects, plants, stars, and planets, all part of nature. We learned about how the natural world stays balanced, and how humans, without intending to, are changing our environment. From these experiences, I gained an avid interest in health and vision.

In my early years, my mother read Adelle Davis's book *Let's Eat Right to Keep Fit.*[16] She gave my father and us children a multivitamin and an extra vitamin C tablet every morning at breakfast. Later, in my twenties, I read several of Adelle Davis's books, learning about carbohydrates, protein, vitamins and nutrients, and how taking vitamin supplements could prevent disease. I hadn't realized it then, but much of Davis's nutritional advice about vitamins and nutrients in food was cutting edge, and was beginning to be retested in nutritional studies. Although nutrition science has progressed in the ensuing years, her original contributions to the field, which helped popularize the idea of nutrition for health, remain significant.

In those early childhood years, I recall reading an article in the *National Geographic* magazine about the national bird, the bald eagle, and the difficulty the species was having due to eggshell thinning. Although many people at the time didn't believe that the pesticide DDT (dichlorodiphenyltrichloroethane) was responsible, and many still do not, it became clear to me that chemicals that persist in the environment can accumulate in biological tissues and can be hazardous to health. I wrote a report about the bald eagle and its fight for survival for my grade-school class. My family also read *Silent Spring* by Rachel Carson,[17] a prescient book about the dangers of pesticides. Not only are synthetic pesticides toxic, they invariably cause the pests (weeds, bugs) to acquire pesticide resistance. A similar resistance can be acquired by bacteria when antibiotics or antibacterial soap are misused.[18] Soon after reading Carson's *Silent Spring,* my family decided that we should stop using the weed poison we had sprayed in our backyard to keep down the dandelions because it was likely killing the worms and other beneficial organisms in the soil as well as the robins that fed on them. We became more aware of the toxic chemicals that get into our food and concentrated in our body, such as mercury in fish, DDT in meat and dairy products, and phthalates in the plastic wrap in meat and cheese packaging, and other dangerous chemicals in the domestic environment.[19] Carson's book sparked a huge new awareness of how industrial society affects the environment, which evolved into the worldwide environmental movement. My mother identified with these strong women who had a scientific interest in health, as she was continually looking for ways to enhance our family's health. As I recollect, these events galvanized my interest in health and nutrition.

Sadly, my mother died of breast cancer in 1969 when I was in college. Although my siblings and I had not been told much about her illness, we had seen her deteriorate for several years, so her death was no surprise. Although it was a tremendous shock, her death helped me understand why she had been so motivated to learn more about nutrition. She had read about vitamins, nutrients, and poisons in the environment because she wanted to survive, and to give us better health so we could survive. It seems likely that the sixteen years she did survive were due at least in part to her healthy diet and vitamin supplements.

When cancer strikes, one tends to question everything, especially anything ingested, for we are what we eat. The same may be true of age-related disease. We naturally want to ask, is it possible that what we have eaten or been exposed to could have been responsible for the disease and the suffering it caused? As it turns out, in the years since my mother's death, health science has made great strides in learning about the dangers of pesticides and chemicals in the environment, and about how adequate amounts of vitamins and nutrients can prevent many diseases such as cancer, heart conditions, and age-related eye diseases. This gave me an earnest motivation to learn about nutrition for health.

I continued my interest in nutrition, reading Linus Pauling's book *Vitamin C and the Common Cold*[20] soon after it was published in 1970, and found it interesting and fairly convincing. Pauling explained why the body needs vitamins, and why our need for vitamin C is much greater than generally recognized. He explained that an adequate dose of vitamin C (3,000 to 10,000 milligrams [mg] per day for many people) can prevent a cold, accelerate recovery from a cold once it starts, and prevent other diseases as well. The book also explained some of the many reasons why the medical profession generally has ignored this treatment. Although vitamin C is very effective and nontoxic even at high doses, many professionals have not paid much attention to the hundreds of studies that have researched and proven its efficacy. Apparently this is because the "vitamin" label seemed to imply (erroneously) that only small doses are required, while vitamin C is most effective at higher doses.

However, I didn't pursue these ideas at that time because I didn't have enough knowledge in biochemistry and physiology to appreciate the truth of what Pauling had been saying. I presumed that Pauling might be correct about the details of vitamin C that he had researched because he was a world famous scientist, having already won two unshared Nobel prizes (the only person ever to do so), and that he knew more than most medical professionals about biochemistry, antioxidants, and the role of vitamin C in the body. But, like many people of that era, I suspected that Pauling might have gotten some of the medical issues wrong or ignored some of the important studies about the effects of vitamins. However, it turned out that Pauling was correct about almost everything he said in his book. We now know, from the many scientific papers and books published since Pauling's book was released in 1970, that vitamin C and other vitamins are helpful in preventing deficiencies that lead to many types of disease.[21] And from the time I read Pauling's book, I took a multivitamin tablet and an extra 1,000mg of vitamin C every day, which I believe has been helpful to my health over the last forty years.

Soon after reading Pauling's book, I read another prescient book, called *Diet for a Small Planet* by Frances Moore Lappé.[22] In that book, Lappé developed a compelling connection between the science of nutrition and the global environmental movement. I learned that much of the world's arable land is used for crops fed to cattle in feed lots. This is an inefficient way to produce protein. More food, along with adequate protein, would be available to people all over the world if we became vegetarian. The book includes a series of tables showing how much protein and other nutrients are in different types of food, the quality of the protein, and the cost of the protein in terms of calories and dollars. It explained that we can get all the nutrition we need from whole grains, vegetables, and fruits much more efficiently than by eating meat. I learned to estimate how much protein was in each type of food and how to enhance its quality by eating foods with complementary proteins, such as grains, legumes (beans and peas), and nuts and seeds. I learned to discern which foods at the supermarket were the best nutritional "buys" (for example, oats, wheat germ, dry beans, collards, kale). I started gardening, and learned to grow my own vegetables, including peas, carrots, beans, tomatoes, broccoli, collards, and kale.

Although nutrition science has made tremendous progress in the last several decades, *Diet for a Small Planet* remains a remarkable exposition of how we can choose to have better nutrition while consuming a fraction of the resources we do now. In the first edition of her book, Lappé explained that, by combining different grains, legumes, nuts, vegetables, and fruits, we can derive a higher-quality diet at less expense than by eating meat. She also detailed her personal journey, through which she became aware of the waste and depletion of resources involved in modern agriculture and meat production. In later versions of the book, Lappé explained that in the ensuing years she learned it is unnecessary to eat a special combination of vegetables to get sufficient protein. For most people, eating an excellent diet of vegetables and fruits will supply enough high-quality protein. This realization has become an important part of modern nutrition science. Overall, the book was important in my education about how the flow of energy in the natural world has been harnessed by humans to grow food. By eating right, we can maximize our efficiency in growing food and minimize our impact on the global environment.

At my breakfast table for the past thirty years I have read the journals *Nature* and *Science,* the two premier basic science journals today. One day about five years ago, while casually browsing through their important articles of general interest, I found an article about vitamin D and how many people are deficient in this essential vitamin. What struck my attention was that the researchers investigating the effects of vitamin D deficiency were trying to determine how much vitamin D was essential for health. Although the clinical experts were saying a dose of 200 to 400 international units (IU) per day would be sufficient, the researchers were saying that 3,000 or even 5,000IU would be optimal. I figured they would know best.

Fascinated, I looked up more articles in medical journals, and learned that vitamin D is only synthesized by the skin from direct exposure to sunlight when the sun is high in the sky. I had assumed I would receive all the vitamin D I needed while I bicycled to work, but I learned that this dosage was completely inadequate in the fall, winter, and spring. And even the dosage I received in the summer was inadequate, because I got to work in the morning before the sun was high in the sky and went home after sunset. Sitting in the sun shining through an ordinary glass window (for example, in a car) may give a tan, but it does not produce vitamin D. Without enough vitamin D, I was risking a multitude of illnesses that would be difficult to detect: cancer, heart disease, seasonal affective disorder, and immune system inadequacy. This very relevant topic and many related ones piqued my interest. To pursue the topic of vitamins and health further, I decided to check on the progress made in the treatment of illness with vitamin C, for I had continued to take 1,000mg with breakfast every day. To my amazement, in a few minutes I found hundreds of recent articles, which seemed overwhelming. So I looked for a review of the topic, and found the book *Ascorbate: The Science of Vitamin* C.[23] It described the latest research on vitamin C and its ability to prevent disease and help the body maintain health. I was fascinated, for evidently the field of vitamin C therapy had progressed steadily since 1970.

Having read the Hickey and Roberts book, I resolved to learn more of the cutting-edge science about vitamins C and D and other essential vitamins and nutrients. I found more books on vitamins C and D[24] and devoured them. Learning more about the importance of vitamin D for the body's utilization of calcium and magnesium, I read Dean's book on magnesium, *The Magnesium Miracle,*[25] and became aware of the importance of correcting a long-term magnesium deficiency that affects many of us. Again

I was amazed by this important information about these easily corrected nutrient deficiencies, well-understood by researchers, but not generally understood or emphasized by medical professionals and most of the people in my daily life. I purchased dozens of copies of these books and sent them to my family and friends, for it was obvious to me that these books could help anyone! One of my friends explained that she didn't have time to read the books. She suggested that I write a "crib sheet" about nutrition, so she and others who were interested but didn't have the time could get the latest nutritional information. I soon found myself reading more books on nutrition. I proceeded to make a list of the most serious nutritional deficiencies most of us have due to our modern diet, and how to prevent them. Thus I was motivated to extend my interest to nutrition from my background studying biochemistry, physiology, and neuroscience.

I ride my bicycle to work every day, and during the winter this tends to stress my lungs, which paid a heavy price when I got sick with a cold. Typically a cold in the winter months would lead to four or five weeks of a heavy cough. This happened to me, as it does to many others, two to three times each year. There is now an abundance of studies showing that vitamin C and other antioxidants are a good way to prevent viral infections and to recover from them faster, especially in the cold.[26] I was motivated to try the regimen of high-dose vitamin C suggested by the books on vitamin C. I started taking 3 grams with every meal, more before going home on my bicycle, and 5 grams before going to bed, totaling 15–20 grams per day, and found that my health improved to the point where I stopped getting colds and flu.[27] When I sensed a viral infection (scratchy throat, headache, tinge of cough), I took 1–3 grams of vitamin C every twenty minutes for several hours until the symptoms abated, then went back to a lower dose. Over the next three years, while I continued to get viruses as they passed through the neighborhood, none of them developed into a full-blown cold or flu. When I finally came down with a more severe cold, with congestion in my nose, it was during a stressful all-day mountain hike in November when I didn't have much vitamin C with me. So I have learned that the dose and the timing is all-important. Vitamin C has helped me to recover from injuries and overexertion, and based on an angiogram that revealed no plaques, I believe it has also contributed to keeping my arteries in good shape.[28]

MY JOB AS A SCIENTIST

A scientist reads and considers the existing scientific literature, develops new scientific questions, and attempts to answer them either by testing hypotheses with direct studies or with careful review of the literature in related fields. In my career studying the structure and function of the retina, I have continually been humbled by the almost incredible complexity and delicacy of the structures of the eye, and also by the hope of millions of people worldwide that studies of the eye can help to prevent and cure blindness. My perspective as a scientist studying the eye's biological function gives me a unique perspective. I have spent thirty years trying to understand how the retina sees the visual world. The progress that I and other scientists like me have made depended heavily on intuition based on research and discoveries in other fields. For example, the physics of molecular diffusion, biophysics of ion channels, biological natural selection, and electronics engineering can be carefully applied to best fit the known facts about the neural circuitry of the retina. In my studies, the scientific questions often came naturally. It was only necessary to read the literature on retinal circuitry with a critical view to find out what was known and what was not known. The hypotheses flowed from that critical reading.

When a hypothesis is generated, testing it is often fairly straightforward. One can readily locate the relevant existing evidence or design new studies to test the hypothesis. In my career I have found that a critical reading of existing literature usually gives strong hints about the answer to the question, which is often the correct one. Once a hypothesis is spelled out clearly along with the supporting evidence, it can then be tested in a variety of ways by scientists around the world. The theory and its testing are welcomed by everyone, no matter what the outcome, because it advances our knowledge in understanding the biological mechanisms. This in turn will help to prevent disease. We now understand much of the signal processing that takes place in the visual pathways of the retina, and we are making progress in understanding why retinal signal processing is necessary. Because there is a long history of knowledge, largely unappreciated, about how nutrition can help to prevent disease, I believe that similar progress can be made in learning how good nutrition can help prevent eye disease.[29]

OUR NEED FOR VITAMINS

Vitamins were first identified by the diseases caused by their deficiency. A person fed a seemingly adequate diet of cooked meat, whole-grain bread, canned vegetables, and dairy products but no fresh fruit or vegetables will succumb in a few months to scurvy, caused by a deficiency of vitamin C. We now know that the active ingredient in raw fruit and vegetables that prevents scurvy is vitamin C (ascorbate), which is very important for every animal species because it is involved in several essential biochemical reactions.[30] It is a necessary cofactor in the synthesis of collagen, which of course is the reason that its deficiency causes scurvy. This means that vitamin C is essential for every organ in the body, to hold together its cells with an extracellular matrix that consists mainly of collagen. It is, therefore, extremely important for the arteries, because their function is to contain blood under pressure. But vitamin C is also one of the main water-soluble antioxidants that circulate in the blood, so it is essential in preventing damage that can quickly destroy the delicate biochemical machinery inside cells. Vitamin C is also important to empower the immune system.[31] Most animals can readily synthesize vitamin C, so for them it is not a vitamin—it's simply one essential component of their normal metabolic pathways. Most animals make a large quantity of vitamin C daily, as much as 10,000mg each day, if their body mass were the same as an adult human.[32] However, the bodies of humans, apes and monkeys, guinea pigs, and fruit-eating bats cannot synthesize vitamin C. We are completely dependent on ingesting an adequate amount of this essential nutrient in our daily meals.

Animals like horses, cows, goats, and antelope, prairie dogs, and buffalo can all survive without vitamin C in their diet. Humans would have a hard time surviving over the winter on their diet of dried grass and water, so it might seem paradoxical that these animals don't need a vitamin that is essential for us. But on further thought we understand why. Their body tissues require vitamin C like ours do, but their diet contains little of it, so their bodies evolved and continued to maintain the metabolic pathways that synthesize it. We know that that early ancestors of primates could make vitamin C because primitive primates, the so-called prosimians (lemurs, loris-es, and galagos), still make this essential biochemical. Our ancestors evolved from later primates in Africa that lived in lush forest and ate generous amounts of vitamin C from fresh leaves and fruits.[33] The DNA (deoxyribonucleic acid, the genetic material in our cells) of most animals codes for enzymes in a biochemical pathway that synthesizes vitamin C. But in the higher primates (tarsiers, monkeys, apes, and humans), the last enzyme in the pathway has mutated, preventing us from synthesizing it.[34] This implies that the mutation was lost in the ancestor common to all these species. Over time, the primate species diverged through natural selection. Those that got enough vitamin C from eating leaves and fruits didn't need any biochemical machinery to synthesize it because they got enough from their diet.

Several hypotheses have been developed about why this mutation was not reversed by natural selection.[35] One hypothesis is that the lack of the ability to make vitamin C could save energy, because its synthesis requires energy, which the body could utilize for other purposes.[36] In any case, it seems likely that some advantage existed for early primates and other animals who lost the ability to make vitamin C, for if there were no advantage, those animals would have died out. A similar loss of the ability to make vitamin C evolved in guinea pigs, capybaras, and fruit-eating bats. They had a diet that included enough vitamin C so their bodies didn't need to make it. The implication is that for millions of years prior to this evolutionary change all animal species could make vitamin C, and only recently in the timeline of history have a few species lost this ability because of their diet.

In a similar way, our need for most other vitamins is thought to have originated from a diet that supplied them. Plants can support their growth by synthesizing biochemicals from minerals and carbon dioxide using energy from the sun, but animals must eat. Some of the biochemicals essential for life, such as proteins, essential oils, and vitamins, were universally available in the diet of primitive animals hundreds of millions of years ago, so over eons their bodies developed a dependency on them. This happened because cells are powerful biochemical factories that require energy and the ingredients to make each chemical cofactor and enzyme. As in the description of vitamin C above, when there is a way to lower the cell's requirement for energy, for example, by using an ingredient readily available in the normal diet of the organism instead of using internal energy to create it, the cell can use that energy for other purposes. The organism as a whole will be healthier and can reproduce faster. Any advantage found by a species that helps one generation give rise to the next will drive the species to maximize that advantage. This is the process of natural selection.

Thus, the rationale behind the body's dependence on all vitamins may be essentially the same in evolutionary terms. Because the bio-chemicals we call vitamins were always present in their diet, our very early ancestors didn't need to synthesize them. As a result they gained a metabolic energy advantage by evolving genetically to become dependent on these biochemicals. From this process, our need for vitamins was born.[37] Most of the vitamins, except vitamin C, are required by all animal species. Vitamin A (5,000 to 10,000IU per day) is essential for the eyes of all animals to regenerate the light-absorbing pigment called "retinal." This vitamin is necessary for vision and for several other important functions in the body. But it is a vitamin because it has been readily available in the diet of most animals from millions of years ago to the present, so animals evolved to depend on these external dietary sources. Similarly, the B and E vitamins are available in the diet of all animals, and vitamin D is synthesized in the skin (10,000IU per day) by direct exposure to midday summer sunlight.

Food Deficiencies Cause Disease

Because vitamins have been available in the diet of animals for eons, the body's dependency on them is a fundamental one. A deficiency of vitamins B, C, D, or E may be difficult to diagnose, because they can cause such a wide range of symptoms. Even more basic are the electrolytes; macronutrients such as sodium, potassium, calcium, and magnesium, and several micronutrients such as iron, zinc, copper, chromium, selenium, and cobalt. Because they are essential to all life and are used widely throughout the body, a deficiency of any of these nutrients can cause wide-ranging problems. For example, because magnesium is utilized in the metabolism of every cell in the body for enzymatic synthesis of DNA, RNA, and protein, a deficiency can give many symptoms, such as high blood pressure, cramps, and asthma. This makes a deficiency difficult to detect in casual observation. Further, many processed foods such as enriched wheat flour or purified sugar and oils contain very little magnesium, so magnesium deficiency is widespread in our population.[38] Unfortunately, the same is true of vitamin C. A nonacute vitamin C deficiency has historically been difficult to detect because it affects every cell in the body. It can be very serious and have far-reaching consequences.[39] Thus, nutrient deficiencies that cause a wide variety of symptoms may be difficult for a medical professional to diagnose—so they are commonly ignored.

A severe deficiency of food and nutrients can have long-lasting effects. For example, the nutrition available to a pregnant woman is extremely important. The nutrients available to the mother, and deficiencies in these nutrients, affect the unborn child's development. During times of famine-for example, in Holland from 1944 to 1945, or in China from 1958 to 1961—children born to mothers who didn't receive sufficient nutrition were affected in many ways. It is currently thought that at least part of this effect is due to an epigenetic modulation of an individual's DNA, which may be passed on to future generations.[40] Children whose mothers were exposed to famine during pregnancy tend to be more obese and tend to have a higher risk of mental illness. A lack of folate in early pregnancy can produce neural tube defects, which may cause a range of physical and neurological disorders, some fatal.[41]

The problem for someone living in the modern world, who tends to rely on processed food, is that the typical modern diet doesn't contain the necessary levels of essential nutrients. Before the industrial revolution, bread was baked from fresh-ground wholewheat flour, and fresh fruits and vegetables were locally grown. But fresh wholewheat flour cannot be stored in open air without refrigeration for more than a few weeks before it starts to spoil. Whole-grain flour contains oils that can go rancid quickly, and it readily supports the growth of mold, so before refrigeration was commonly available, white flour was prized as being safer. In the late 1800s it was discovered that steel rolling mills could efficiently remove the wheat grain's bran and germ.[42] Millers found this dramatically increased the shelf life of their flour, making white flour widely available for the masses.

The unfortunate result was that epidemics of dietary deficiency diseases became common in the 1890s and early 1900s. We now know that the deficiencies of essential nutrients that hinder growth of fungus and mold on white flour also hinder human health. A few decades later, it was discovered that wheat bran and germ, the parts of the kernel removed in the refining process, could prevent the deficiency diseases when added to the diet. This led to the discovery of the missing essential nutrients. Heroic laboratory investigations during the early 1900s revealed the identity of these essential nutrients,[43] which were eventually named "vitamins." Enriched flour helped relieve the vitamin deficiency epidemics because some of the essential nutrients were added after refining. Unfortunately, however, the typical enriched flour is incomplete, because it is deficient in essential nutrients such as magnesium and vitamin E. The same loss of essential nutrients in the refining process is also true of most other refined foods, such as oil and sugar. The more refined a product like olive oil or cane sugar becomes, the less other essential nutrients it contains.

Further, the commercial process of growing food in our modern society has evolved to the point where much of the food we eat is grown on mechanized farms that depend on refined chemicals for the fertility of their soil. The problem with this is that often the fertilizers applied do not replace some of the essential nutrients, such as magnesium, selenium, and other trace elements, required in our diet. Over a period of several decades, the normal electrolyte content of the soil required by common plant crops such as peppers and tomatoes becomes depleted. Further, modern cultivars of grains have reduced the amount of minerals they contain.[44] Thus the commercial produce that is trucked to our markets today has lower levels of vitamins and nutrients than fifty years ago.[45]

This raises the question of how we can get the nutrients our bodies need. Organic farming is one way, for organic produce tends to have fewer pesticides and more nutrients, including magnesium and vitamin C, than ordinary produce from agribusiness.[46] Local farming and farmers markets have recently become more popular in many states. The advantage of locally-grown produce is that it requires less fossil fuel than produce trucked across the country, and in season it tends to be fresher with higher level of nutrients. At least one nationwide retail chain-store has decided to sell local organic produce at low cost so bargain hunters can also have good nutrition. The mayor's office of Philadelphia, Pennyslvania, supports a Greenworks program that aims to start and help maintain new neighborhood gardens, sc every resident is within a ten-block walk of fresh produce in season. These efforts can benefit everyone who wants to eat a healthier diet. This is especially true of those who wish to have more healthier eyes, for as you will see below, dark green leafy vegetables may be almost a panacea for eye diseases.

In the mid-twentieth century, vitamin supplements were developed to supply missing nutrients, Multivitamin supplements were designed to prevent common, easily recognized nutrient deficiencies, Medical nutrition boards were set up to determine the average amount of each nutrient a person require to prevent a specific symptom of deficiency. An upper limit was also determined for children and adults, so the safety of the supplement could be assured. The amount of nutrients thought to be suitable for the "average" person were then included in a convenient tablet.[47] Thus, multivitamin tablets, because they readily eliminate many nutrient deficiencies, can be an important factor in health.

But the facts about nutrients aren't quite so simple. People who take a given quantity of a nutrient, such as water-soluble vitamin C or fat-soluble vitamin D, often have a threefold difference or more of the nutrient in their blood levels. The reason is that digestion, absorption, distribution, and utilization of nutrients by the body vary greatly. A large person (200 pounds) will need more nutrients such as vitamin C (10–20 grams a day) or vitamin D (7,000–10,000IU a day) than someone smaller. Because it is important for the body to get the right concentration of these nutrients, the actual amount you need to take varies according to your body weight. Thus, the doses of nutrients are often given normalized to body weight. For example, vitamin C is often taken at 30–100mg per kilogram daily (15–50mg per pound daily). Those who are overweight, with a higher fraction of fat in their bodies, may need even more vitamin D (10,000–15,000IU daily or more) to maintain an adequate blood level.

The blood levels of fat-soluble nutrients like vitamins A, D, and E rise and fall slowly because the body's fat tends to absorb and regulate them. The half-life of vitamin D in the body (the time it takes for the concentration to drop by 50 percent) is several weeks to months.[48] For this reason the level of vitamin D takes a long time to rise in the body's tissues, and also a long time to fall. This "time constant" is not identical among individuals, but varies depending on several factors such as the relative absorption efficiency and the body mass index (how much fat the body contains).

The opposite is true of water-soluble vitamins such as vitamin C and many of the B vitamins. These have a short half-life in the body. For B vitamins this is typically less than several days, and for vitamin C it can be as short as four to eight hours.[49] Their level rises quickly in the bloodstream, but then falls quickly too. These water-soluble vitamins should be taken at least once or more per day, preferably several times in divided doses, to maintain a high average level. One might imagine that it is futile to try to raise the body's level of vitamin C because it gets excreted quickly, and the uptake mechanism in the kidneys for vitamin C gets saturated at a low level. But during the time it transits the bloodstream, vitamin C does its job for the body, preventing oxidative damage and asserting its necessary role in the synthesis of collagen.[50] So high doses of vitamin C (3,000–10,000mg daily) are beneficial. The eye has a heavy requirement for vitamin C. Every time a dose of vitamin C is taken, its blood level rises quickly allowing the eye to take up more vitamin C to prevent disease.

Further, each person's requirement for nutrients is based on their individual needs, which originate in their personal genetics, their exposure to environmental toxins and disease, and their daily levels of stress. This was shown in animal studies on vitamin C in guinea pigs, one of the few animals that, like us, cannot make vitamin C in their bodies.[51] The guinea pigs were given a diet without vitamin C, and then different groups of animals were maintained for more than a year on different amounts of supplemental vitamin C. The study showed that vitamin C on average was beneficial for weight gain, but that individual animals varied greatly in their response and need for vitamin C. Some individual animal given no vitamin C developed symptoms of scurvy, but survived nevertheless. Some animals did not seem to benefit from a large supplement of vitamin C, but other animals got a huge benefit. The study concluded that some individuals are better able to deal with a vitamin-C deficiency than others, possibly because their bodies can synthesize or regenerate a little vitamin C. The same variable dependency on vitamin C is also true of primates and humans, and it is also true for every other essential nutrient required by the body. Our nutrient needs vary widely among individuals.[52]

Each essential nutrient has a different route into the body, and a different use by the body. Some nutrients, for example, water-soluble vitamin C and many of the B vitamins, are easily absorbed but also easily lost in the urine. These water-soluble vitamins require special biochemical uptake pathways in the kidneys to keep them from being excreted. However, some nutrients require a more complex apparatus just to get them absorbed. For example, although we need only a tiny amount of vitamin B_{12}—just a few micrograms (mcg) per day)—we need a special "binding protein" secreted into the gut, and a special "transporter protein" to take it up into our tissues.[53] Also, the tissues of higher primates have special transporters that allow red blood cells to take up oxidized vitamin C and reduce it back to its original active form. It is then released again to the bloodstream, recycling this essential nutrient to some extent.[54] It is also known that vitamin E can be recycled back to its active form by vitamin C.[55] Many combinations of nutrients are synergistic in this way.

To find the most effective treatment, one would like to follow scientific principles. The term for this is to use "evidence-based" treatments. That means we try to understand the results of modern health studies and take the treatment that has worked the best. The next chapters will give an overview of the evidence that adequate levels of vitamins and nutrients can help to prevent ailments, including many age-related eye diseases. While pharmaceutical companies make their profits from drugs, it has become clear to evidence-based medicine that nutrition plays an important role in preventing and treating high blood pressure, heart disease, diabetes, cancer, and many other diseases of modern society. This is captured in the term "nutraceutical;" which means foods or nutrition that can take the place of or enhance the use of pharmaceuticals.[56] Because heart disease, high blood pressure, diabetes, and many other whole-body ailments can directly affect the eye, the nutritional prevention and treatment of these diseases is of interest to anyone with eye disease.

With modern technology, it is possible to measure the blood levels of different nutrients and metabolic products and also to characterize portions of anyone's genome relevant to their utilization of these nutrients. This has spurred the development of "nutrigenomics," the study of how nutrition affects gene expression, and how differences in gene expression affect the absorption, utilization, and thus the need for nutrients in the body.[57] Many large food corporations are interested in pursuing this type of science, because there are profits to be made in optimizing the intake of nutrients for individuals, depending on their genetic makeup, age, or relevant disease.[58] Pharmaceutical companies have spent millions on way to analyze the genome for problems that cause disease, because this allows them to develop drugs that may help. But this genetic information has made it clear that, because individual differences in our genetic makeup affect our need for nutrients, optimal nutrition will be important in our search for health.[59] Thus it may soon be possible to for an individual to focus on certain nutrients that are critical given their genetic make-up.[60] I believe this is exactly what Linus Pauling had in mind when he coined the term "orthomolecular medicine."[61]

Age-Related Deficiencies

Older people have all the issues with nutrients described above, but in addition have special difficultie1 obtaining enough of them.[62] When we are young and growing fast, our robust appetites supply enough nutrients for growth. However, many teenagers and young adults have not learned to eat well, and their diet often lacks essential nutrients such as vitamins C and D and magnesium. Young bodies can live with this for a few years, but as we age, getting enough nutrients becomes much more difficult, for several reasons.

Aging tissue needs extra nutrients to repair damage done over decades of wear and tear. Every time we get cut or bruised or get a severe cold or flu, the immune system sends special cells and biochemicals to the site, generating more blood flow, which causes inflammation. The body sends fibroblast stem cells to the site of inflammation, and they repair the damage.[63] However, this ability is contingent upon having a sufficient activity of stem cells. An insufficient amount of essential nutrients can slow this healing process.

Further, as we age, many of us become more sedentary, so our need for food declines. But our appetite tends to continue unabated, so we tend to put on weight. When attempting to reduce their weight, many people try to eat less, but they continue to eat the same customary nutrient-poor food. One can reduce calorie intake by eating smaller portions at each meal, but this also reduces the amount of nutrients—at a time when the body needs more nutrients. Older people commonly have several nutrient deficiencies, which can cause many types of impairments.[64] Thus, as we age, to stay healthy we must typically focus on eating a better diet that includes a higher level of nutrients.[65]

Nutrient deficiencies can cause many serious age-related diseases, such as heart disease, strokes, arthritis, neurological problems, dementia, and many eye problems.[66] When someone has eaten a nutrient-poor diet for several decades, the deficiencies compound in several ways. First, the body can accumulate a deficit of a nutrient. For example, a magnesium deficit is very common due to the modern diet of processed foods. Such a deficit is difficult to diagnose using a blood test, because the level of magnesium in the bloodstream stays relatively constant even with a prolonged deficit.[67] The bones hold most of the body's magnesium, and they function as a magnesium reservoir. So, when the body needs magnesium, for example after a day of vigorous exercise, it takes magnesium from the bones to fulfill its needs. This is okay when the diet averaged over several days contains enough magnesium to replace the amount removed. But when there is a continual long-term lack of magnesium in the diet, the result is a deficit that can build up in the body over many years, leading to a continual depletion of magnesium required for normal function throughout the body.[68]

But there is a worse problem associated with a lack of nutrition in old age. Many older people choose not to eat raw fruits and vegetables that contain a lot of fiber. These foods are important sources of nutrients. This bland diet presents the aging body with a further challenge: It can limit the body's ability to absorb nutrients. Proper digestion requires a robust supply of nutrients to generate the enzymes, bile, and hydrochloric acid, necessary for breaking down food into molecules. A deficiency in these nutrients hinders digestion by the stomach and intestines—which accelerates the deficiency. Thus, as we age, our bodies need more nutrients, but for many reasons we tend to get less. All of these factors imply that better nutrition can prevent age-related diseases.

In order to understand the relatively high incidence of age-related diseases, Ames[69] hypothesized that eons ago, when our distant ancestors were afflicted by famines, their bodies were stressed by vitamin and nutrient deficiencies. Many nutrients are required for several functions in the body, for example, basic energy production, preventing oxidative damage, and combating age-related disease. But energy metabolism took precedence over longer-term functions such as maintenance of arteries.[70] Thus, long ago, animals' biochemical pathways evolved to utilize the scarce nutrients preferentially for energy production at the expense of the body's other longer-term needs. Ames hypothesized that the enzymes directly involved in energy production were modified by evolution to have a greater affinity for the essential nutrients. Thus the nutrients became monopolized by energy production. However, this tended to prevent the nutrients from being utilized for long-term maintenance functions of the body, such as preventing oxidative stress, heart disease, and cancer.[71]

This "triage" hypothesis can explain the high incidence of age-related diseases such as heart disease, cancer, and diabetes when nutrition is poor.[72] Although this hypothesis will require many years of study to be fully tested, it matches what is known about the risk factors for long-term disease, such as DNA damage and inflammation. When a nutrient-poor diet causes an accumulation of damage in tissues, a cell's mitochondria cannot function as well to generate energy, which leads to further accumulation of damage. The reason is that the cell requires energy to defend itself against oxidative stress.[73] We will discuss this topic further in Chapter 3.

The Effect of Nutrient Deficiency on Eye Health

Poor nutrition has a direct impact on eye health, and this deterioration becomes more acute within the aging eye. For example, a diet insufficient in magnesium is thought to contribute to glaucoma, because this deficiency typically raises blood pressure. An insufficiency in antioxidants is thought to contribute to the gradual deterioration of eye tissues in glaucoma, macular degeneration, and retinitis pigmentosa. A lack of antioxidants in the eye tissues can accelerate normal wear-and-tear from our daily lives, limiting the ability of the tissues to maintain themselves. The consequence is that the eye tissues slowly degrade and lose their normal ability to function. A lack of B vitamins can cause many problems in blood vessels and in tissues throughout the body,[74] including in the eye. Another example is the level of vitamin C in the bloodstream. Vitamin C is necessary for the production of collagen. When vitamin C is absent, tissues throughout the body, such as capillaries of the retina, cannot be maintained because the collagen they contain becomes weak and easily torn.[75] By eating healthier, it is possible to prevent or reverse these types of age-related diseases. This topic will be discussed in Chapter 8.

CHAPTER 2

HOW SCIENCE LEARNS: STUDIES OF TREATMENTS

Over recorded history, knowledge about our bodies and our world has developed as one of the most important benefits of civilization. Science developed from ordinary people wondering about the natural world and asking simple questions, which they tried to answer in terms that would be understandable and convincing to others. In ancient times, this was historically the role of village shamans, religious leaders, and, eventually, philosophers. After the appearance of books and once reading became widespread, the questions raised by philosophers inspired a new enthusiasm for learning about the natural world. During the Age of Enlightenment from the 1600s to the 1800s, science became a separate vocation that called upon reason rather than dogma to explain the natural world's wonders. Over the past two centuries, science (including physics, chemistry, and biology) has developed into the study of the mechanisms of the natural world, and is widely credited with providing a basis for progress in health and the treatment of disease. People in many countries have discovered, by trial and error, combinations of fruits and vegetables that cure disease. Modern science can improve on this method using an objective approach based on our knowledge of biochemistry.

SCIENTIFIC QUESTIONS AND HYPOTHESES

Several standard paradigms exist for developing scientific knowledge. Generally, as more knowledge about a topic such as a disease, biochemical pathway, or vitamin becomes available, it raises new questions about the mechanism(s) responsible for what was observed. A hypothesis, or theory, is developed that contains an essential concept attempting to explain what is already known through its proposed mechanisms. The central paradigm, or framework, of modern science is that it is "hypothesis-driven." The hypothesis is tested with data from controlled experiments. If the hypothesis explains more of the observed results than previous theories, it is accepted as a working theory and assimilated into scientific knowledge. This assimilation may take years, or in some cases, decades or centuries. For example, the discovery by James Lind that scurvy could be treated with citrus fruits in the diet (that contain vitamin C) was not recognized for nearly fifty years by the British Navy. It took another two centuries for vitamin C to be discovered and its use in preventing common health problems to be understood.[76]

Yet, the assimilation of new knowledge about vitamins can be almost immediate. For example, over the last decade, medical researchers clarified the role of vitamin D in health, redefining its importance. They showed that it is necessary for the body, not only to cure and prevent bone diseases like rickets at a dose of 400IU per day, but as a powerful hormone for the entire body, important in preventing many types of cancer.[77] Much higher doses of vitamin D supplements, equivalent to the approximately 10,000 international units (IU) that we can get in the summer by sufficient midday sun exposure, are now advised by many doctors and nutritionists. The new knowledge, now widely available in books, the media, and on the Web, was made available to the public fairly quickly.

When competing hypotheses about a disease or its cure are developed they are tested against existing hypotheses by comparing the available data, and the differences resolved either by discarding hypotheses or by modifying them. Often several competing hypotheses are driven by "interest groups" of scientists working on different aspects of a disease. The scientific question asked by the interest groups may differ, and as a result they will have different outlooks that emphasize different aspects of treatment for the disease. For example, when presented with someone who has an age-related eye disease such as glaucoma, macular degeneration, or retinitis pigmentosa, ophthalmologists typically focus on treating the acute symptoms of the diseases, hoping to preserve the patient's vision. In a study of these diseases, the eye doctor might ask scientific questions about how the eye disease progresses when treated with a drug.[78]

An orthomolecular nutritionist/physician presented with the same patient would likely take a different approach, emphasizing the prevention of the age-related disease and its reversal using adequate amounts of essential nutrients. As in the story recounted early in Chapter 1 about the woman going blind, the nutritionist would likely recommend a healthy diet along with supplements, individualized to the patient's needs; for example, generous servings of leafy green vegetables, sprouts, fruits, whole grains, yogurt, a small amount of meat, vitamin C to bowel tolerance (2,000–10,000 milligrams per day), vitamin D (5,000–10,000IU per day), vitamin E with tocopherols and tocotrienols (400–1,200IU per day), zinc(50milligrams), selenium(100micrograms), copper(2milligrams), magnesium(300milligrams), and calcium (500 milligrams). The nutritionist would work with the patient's doctors to optimize the treatment and minimize possible detrimental interactions with any drug therapy given. For a young adult patient with early signs of the disease, the nutritionist would advise getting on the healthy diet immediately, instead of waiting until the age of sixty for the age-related disease to be treated.

A study based on this principle of health treatment would obviously ask a different scientific question than the one based on the study of a drug. The results of the two types of study might be very different, because how a person reacts to a drug, with its potential side effects, is likely to differ from how a person reacts to an excellent diet and optimal combinations of nutrients—and the conclusions would likely diverge. The decision about which treatment works better would depend on how the studies were done and the scientific questions that were asked. If the question is what is the best way to prevent age-related eye disease and attempt to reverse it, the answer may very well be to get on an excellent diet, stop smoking, get adequate exercise and sleep, wear a wide-brimmed hat and dark glasses when in the sunlight for many hours, and take an adequate level of supplements.[79] Note, however, that standard medical treatment using drugs and orthomolecular medicine are not necessarily at odds. Good nutrition will invariably benefit those who are taking drugs to treat a disease.[80]

OBJECTIVITY AND ETHICS OF HEALTH STUDIES

In the scientific study of health, a major concern is the objectivity of the experiments, because our lives cannot be experimentally controlled like chemicals in a test tube. People have preferences and subtle differences in their daily lives that complicate the analysis of study results. Further, health studies must be designed to address concerns about ethical issues. Ideally, patients with serious illness should never be given a treatment in a study that is already known to be less than optimally effective. If the treatment being tested is already known to be effective, then it would be unethical not to provide it to all the patients in the study who would benefit from it. The patients must always be informed about what the study is testing and about the possible side effects, and with this knowledge they sign a consent form.[81] However, this is not always possible, because to fully inform a patient about the treatment they receive might bias the outcome. And it would be unethical to give different treatments where one is known to be less effective, even though the purpose of the study is to test hypotheses about the treatment's suspected benefits.

Other issues can make the results of health studies unreliable. To test the safety and efficacy of a new treatment, the therapy may be given to a relevant population, say, a group selected with a particular eye disease. Some of that group, however, may read about medicine and nutrition and eat a healthy diet. The effect of the treatment in these people may differ from its effect in others who eat a less healthy diet. The differing lifestyles of these two subgroups, if not identified, can affect the study's statistical outcome. Further, a patient should always have the option to drop out of the study. A common reason for dropping out, specified in the consent forms, is that the patient develops any of a variety of acute symptoms related to the study, such as requiring hospitalization and further specific treatments for the disease. This can further bias the study, because the treatment may have affected the patient's symptoms in either a positive or negative way that may not be fully taken into account in the study data after they drop out. The results of a health study can also get confused when individuals in the study group, who were selected because they have a particular disease (for example, heart disease) have other related diseases, such as emphysema, cancer, or eye disease, that have a common cause such as smoking or drinking alcohol. In this case, the common cause for all of these diseases can bias the study's conclusions. These problems are ubiquitous in health studies. The objectivity of the study can be affected by how the patients are treated for the primary disease being studied or other related diseases.

Subjective Effects

Doctors learned centuries ago that when patients were given a treatment without any active ingredients specific for their condition, they very often reported improvement in their symptoms. The effect is thought to be related to the patients' expectation of improvement, and is called the "placebo effect." It can be important in relieving psychologically relevant symptoms such as pain. The placebo effect is thought to be caused by the brain through autonomic control of body functions such as the heart rate, respiration rate, body temperature, immune system, and organs of the body such as the liver and gut, which are responsible for many aspects of health and recovery from disease. Any substance given to the patient for treatment can in principle induce this type of subjective improvement, which may be an important part of the patient's recovery. Or it may confound the treatment, making it more difficult. Other subjective effects can originate from apparent bias in the doctor's investigation and treatment of a patient's symptoms. A doctor may be biased in different ways toward patients, based on their symptoms, gender, or lifestyle. Doctors try to minimize such bias, of course, and for serious diseases often agonize over decisions about the best type of treatment. One way to minimize this type of subjective physician bias in a study is to analyze the effect of a treatment on a large group of patients. Then the data from the outcome of the experiment is averaged, thereby reducing the bias toward individuals. Such a test of a treatment is called a "clinical trial" and of all studies it is the most basic.

Random Effects

In any health study, one of the main concerns is variability among the subjects. There are several reasons for variability. Every individual has a unique set of genes, and these genes are expressed (are used) in the body to a different degree, depending on the environmental stresses and nutrition available during development as an unborn fetus and throughout infancy and childhood. Also, every individual has a different diet that supplies different amounts of nutrients, and these nutrients are absorbed differently by the individual's gut. Further, each individual is subjected to unique daily stresses and exposure to environmental toxins, bacteria, and viruses-and we all have different paths through each day and through our lives. If you were given nutritious food as a child, you are more likely to grow up healthy, but this will depend on your exposure to bacteria, how they colonize your gut, and how they affect your ability to absorb nutrients. For example, recent research shows that if you are exposed to sufficient sunlight as a young child, your risk of many adult diseases is reduced. But usually it is not possible to discover the opposite; that is, to know exactly what in an individual's history was the cause of a particular disease. Although in theory each of the multitude of effects can be tracked down, there are usually too many factors in an individual's life that affect their health to allow a doctor to know the precise cause of a health problem. For this reason, when any group of people is studied, although they may have many similarities in their patterns of health, there are invariably "random effects" that cannot be easily explained from what is known about the individuals in the group.

The theory of random effects states that the standard deviation—that is, the expected variability in the number of random events in a group—is proportional to the square root of the average number of events. For example, if each person in a group eats on the average 14 carrots per week, and if the motivation to eat them was completely random for each person, the actual numbers would vary according to a random distribution with the standard deviation equal to 3.7. In other words, although the actual number of carrots eaten would be random and thus could be any number, most of the people in the group would eat between ten and eighteen carrots, and only a few would eat less than six or more than twenty-two. When the group of people is large, it is fairly straightforward to estimate the range of this variability in the overall population. However, if the sample is small, the estimates of the average and its range of variability (within+/-one standard deviation of the average) are less accurate. For example, in the example above, the average rate in a household of four people is eight carrots per day. The expected random variability is 2.8, that is, between a low of five carrots and a high of eleven carrots. If two households picked at random are studied, commonly one will have a lower occurrence of carrots eaten, for example, five carrots, and the other will have a larger number, say ten carrots. If the variability is thought to be random, small differences in the numbers of events between groups will have no meaning because they are expected as an effect of random fluctuation.

The same reasoning applies to any type of event, such as the rate of a disease, or the rate of cure by a treatment. Although any rate of occurrence of a disease is possible, when the differences between groups in a study are less than what is expected from random variability, one must question whether the differences are meaningful. If the difference in the rate of occurrence between groups is twice or three times the expected variability, it is usually pretty safe to say the difference originates from a specific cause and is not just a random event. This is not always true, because a random event is impossible to predict, but when the difference in the rate is close to the expected random variability, one can only say it isn't very meaningful. To achieve a more meaningful result in treating a disease, it is useful to study larger groups or a more effective treatment. Then one can decide whether the treatment is effective, based on how the variability compares with purely random probability. A major challenge for health studies is to disentangle these effects.

Observational Studies

To get an objective measure of the effect of a treatment, health studies commonly categorize a population into two or more groups, or "cohorts;" one that was given a treatment and the other, called the "control group;" that was either given no treatment or a similar but ineffective treatment (a placebo). In some studies, there may also be "normal" and "disease" groups, which may be further split into two groups, treated and untreated, to better discern and compare the effect of treatment. When the health status of the groups is observed but they are not given any experimental treatment, it is called an "observational study." Any treatment or disease condition the participants already have is thus already known to them. When a sufficiently large population is studied, the study can identify the benefit of treatment, even if it is small, by comparing and subtracting the results obtained by observing the two groups. When a control group takes an ineffective treatment, it may obtain some benefit based on the placebo effect, but this factor can be reduced by including other normal groups without disease in the study. The results from each group are then averaged and the results studied for the true effect of the treatment.

However, the observational method cannot completely eliminate the placebo effect, nor can it eliminate subjective physician bias. The reasons are several. A group without disease may react to a treatment or placebo differently than a group with the disease, complicating the comparison of results. Further, the selection and treatment of the study groups is susceptible to subjective bias in both patient and doctor. For example, in observational studies where the patients know what treatment they have received, attentive patients may notice whether or not their treatment is causing an improvement and may compensate in their lifestyle without necessarily being aware they are doing so. They may change their exercise, level of daily stress, or diet, for example. This can cause a change in health status that is difficult to track. And a doctor may unwittingly select healthier patients for a particular group, either the treated or control group, causing unreliable results.

Double-Blind and Randomized Controlled Trials

In an "interventional study," the administrators of the study decide which participants get the treatment. To lessen patient bias, the participants are not told whether they are receiving the treatment being tested or the placebo. However, this cannot prevent the attentive patient from discovering the efficacy of their treatment, especially when the doctor presenting the treatment knows which group the patient is in. There is always the possibility that the doctor unintentionally gives the patient some clue about the treatment. Thus, in studies where the doctor knows which treatment is being presented, it is still possible that interactions between patient and doctor are biased, causing unreliable results. To prevent this possibility, the study can be "double-blind." In this type of study neither the doctor presenting the treatment nor the patient know which treatment has been given. Administrators of the study make the selections of treatments, but don't see or interact with the patients. Even in this case, however, it is still possible that the selection of the study groups (treatment versus placebo) is biased. To remove any potential subjective bias in studies of diseases or their treatment, the selection of patients for the study is made at random. This is called a randomized controlled trial (RCT). Each patient in the study is randomly chosen to be in one of several study groups, but neither the patient nor attending doctor is told which one, to prevent subjective bias.

The power of an RCT is that any significant effect of the interventional treatment must have originated in some way from the difference between the treated and untreated groups. Although a significant effect from such a study does not imply the treatment has directly caused the effect, it does suggest a path of causality. Like other types of studies, the RCT is prone to random effects, so it may give spurious results. As described above, it is necessary to study a large population to get rid of random effects. Thus, large double-blind randomized controlled trials, where neither patient nor presenting physician knows the patient's study group or treatment, are widely considered the "gold standard" of health research, because they can eliminate or reduce many of the confounding effects in other types of studies. But not even the RCT can always give a clear answer to a simple scientific question.

Positive Versus Negative Results: Proportionality

In any scientific study, one hopes that there will be an obvious effect of the treatment that clearly shows a difference between the patient study groups. If the groups are large, the individual differences between patients are averaged and thus ignored in favor of the treatment's overall effect. However, in studies of complex issues like health, the results often do not show any overall effect. This can happen for several reasons. It is possible that the scientific question was not correctly tested, the groups were not large enough to provide a good average free from random variations, or the treatment was ineffective due to a confounding issue such as a related disease or lifestyle in the population being tested. For example, in a study testing the effect of nutrition or drug treatment on the onset of glaucoma, if some patients have high blood pressure, a likely risk factor for glaucoma, they may know this and actively try to reduce their blood pressure with proper diet and reduction in stress. However, other patients in the study who don't have high blood pressure may continue with a more stressful lifestyle. Or, worse, some patients who have high blood pressure but are unaware of the consequences may continue with a stressful lifestyle and a poor diet. If these effects are not taken into account in the study, their effect on the treatment of the study may confound its results. To reduce these effects, many studies use several study groups given treatment in different proportions. The rationale is that any meaningful results should be related to the amount of treatment. If a stronger treatment is more effective, then when a weaker treatment shows no obvious result, at least this is consistent. However, if both a weaker and a stronger treatment are effective, it is possible that there is a confounding bias factor in the treatment or the lifestyles of the study groups, or possibly the treatment is so effective that it could be given at a lower dose. But if both weaker and stronger treatment are ineffective, one needs to pause and rethink the treatment and the scientific question.

Correlation and Causality

As described above, the random-controlled trial is widely held to be the best way to establish facts about a medical treatment. An RCT with a very clear conclusion is supposed to show causality. An observational study is only able to show a correlation. The term *correlation* may sound highly mathematical, but it need not be a mathematical concept. It means, simply, that when one result appears along with a second one, there is some relationship. The two results could be, say, beautiful flowers growing exceptionally well in a garden and bountiful vegetables ripening nearby. When they occur together, they are correlated. If someone asks why, we might naively say, maybe the flowers' presence near the vegetables caused the vegetables to grow bigger and tastier. This is an example of a hypothesis about causality that originates from a correlated result. Yet, gardeners would tell us that these correlated results of gardening are likely caused by good soil, watering, and care of the plants.

This, in scientific terms, is a hypothesis about the cause of the correlation-in this case, that the correlated results are a consequence of a mechanism in common. In an interventional RCT, the correlation between the treatment and the effect is often considered to indicate causality. But the path of causality can be long, with many correlated effects that can be very difficult to identify.

A big part of our lives is related to tracking correlations, which can be useful even if they don't lead us to the cause. An analogy is the search for a good source of food. If we try a new restaurant and find excellent food, we may be more likely to eat there again. Our expectation is that the quality of the restaurant's food is correlated over time. Using this approach, to find a supply of food is a matter of tracking correlations. An interesting example of this is how a bacterium, a tiny one-celled organism too small for us to see with the naked eye, can find a raisin dropped into a bucket of water without any sense of sight, direction, or knowledge about where it is. The bacterium has an exquisite sense of the amount (concentration) of sugar or other nutrients in a liquid environment, and it can swim for a few seconds in one direction. How does this enable it to find the raisin? Amazingly, it can locate the exact source of sugar simply by remembering how much food it sensed a short time ago.[82] If the concentration of sugar doesn't increase, the bacterium tumbles randomly every few seconds to head off in a new direction.

If the concentration of sugar increases, the bacterium tumbles less often, so it tends to head in the direction of increasing sugar, and eventually it finds the raisin and has a feast. This is an example of a correlation. The bacterium makes use of the fact that the source of sugar is correlated over space due to diffusion through the water, which causes the concentration of sugar it senses to be correlated in time. The more sugar it senses, the closer it is to the raisin. However, the bacterium doesn't "know" where the food is. It can only swim blindly in random directions, and it has no theory for where the food is nor the direction in which it should swim to get there. The moral of this story is that in a complex world or in a well-intentioned health study, correlations in our observations can be very helpful, but they don't always lead to knowledge about the cause.

In some health studies, nutrient supplements show a small increase in disease risk, or they may show a decrease in disease risk. Others show no effect of supplements at all, even with large study groups in double-blind randomized trials. Many people would assume that these studies are conclusive because they were conceived and performed with the best scientific methods. However, knowledge in science, especially health science, comes from understanding causality. When a new hypothesis is tested and is found to explain the results of a study, it may be tentatively accepted, but if in further tests it is found to be incorrect, science must sometimes find an alternative hypothesis that fits the data better. If an RCT can identify a strong correlation between a treatment and a benefit, this can suggest causality and may help to develop a strong hypothesis about the disease mechanism, the mechanism for the benefit, and how to best improve treatment. But this conclusion should only be considered valid for the specific experimental question considered and may be difficult to generalize. If an RCT can identify a weak correlation between a treatment and a benefit, it may help to further develop hypotheses, but there will always be some uncertainty about the result.

A weak correlation can be caused by many factors, including random variation in an inadequate population size or correlations between the lifestyle of patients in the study and their diseases. When two diseases have a similar origin—for example, glaucoma and heart disease, both related to high blood pressure—this can affect the results of a study positively or negatively. The reason is that in many studies of serious disease, for ethical considerations an acute symptom or hospitalization dictates that the study should stop considering that patient. When a subject is removed from the study because of a heart attack, this will influence the statistical risk of the remaining participants because they are less likely to have acute heart problems, which may cause them, statistically, to be either more or less likely to get glaucoma. If high blood pressure is the primary cause of both diseases, those who have acute heart problems may be most at risk for glaucoma, and thus the remaining participants will have a statistically lower risk for glaucoma. If the cause of glaucoma in some patients is heavily affected by other factors, a treatment that lessens acute heart problems may keep more of the original participants in the study, and thus cause a higher statistical risk for glaucoma. Thus, many complex interactions exist between correlated symptoms and diseases that even a carefully designed RCT cannot easily untangle.

A lack of correlation is even more difficult to determine, because a negative result does not have the same explanatory power as a positive one. An obvious reason for negative results is random variation, for if the effect of treatment is too weak (for example, a dose is too low) it may be completely obscured by random effects.[83] But a negative effect can also be caused by the wrong scientific question, the wrong hypothesis, or an unexpected correlation. In a simplistic analogy, if you look for kangaroos in Kansas, or ginseng in Georgia, but don't find any, you may not be looking in the right habitat, or even the right country! But without a theory, the negative result does not give much assurance that what you're searching for doesn't exist. Therefore an RCT studying a health treatment with a negative result must be interpreted in the context of the diseases and lifestyles of the study groups, and all the possible correlations and random variations that might affect the results. Although some correlations can be explicitly taken into account in the analysis of the study's results, this is not always possible.

HEALTH STUDIES ARE COMPLEX AND EXPENSIVE

The bottom line is that health studies are full of complexities that can bias their results, so they require careful planning. They are usually expensive because they require the services of medical professionals typically over a period of many years.[84] The scientific questions asked by a health study, to test a treatment and its dose, must not only be relevant, but must also test an effect that is robust enough to overwhelm random variability. Often, the best evidence about a treatment comes from large RCTs that study several control groups; for example, split into untreated normal, untreated disease, treated normal, treated disease. These groups can be split further when the treatment is given at several doses to check for proportionality. But RCTs are not always appropriate, for example, when the treatment is obvious to the patient, or when it is unethical not to supply a treatment.

Observational studies are sometimes the only way to derive important health information, and they can be very powerful.[85] For example, an observational study can follow people already given a treatment or a drug to see how different aspects of daily life affect the outcome. Or, a rare disease can be studied by searching for correlated factors in the lives of those affected. For example, when a combination of nutrients, such as vitamin D, calcium, and magnesium, is thought likely to provide a benefit for a clinical condition such as high blood pressure but there is not enough evidence to initiate a large RCT, doctors may interview a group of patients with or without the condition, asking about their intake of the nutrients to informally test the benefit. Then, if the expected benefit is found, the nutrients can be tested more thoroughly alone or in different combinations in a larger health study. However, because large studies are expensive, they are often initiated by pharmaceutical corporations that are testing new drug candidates and can afford to set up and run the test. An obvious problem for initiating a large health study to test the effect of nutritional treatments is that these treatments are usually not patentable. Thus, large pharmaceutical corporations generally do not support big, expensive studies of vitamins, nutrients, and orthomolecular treatments.

Participants in a health study and any patients that have a disease want and deserve to know the best treatment as quickly as possible, so there is tremendous pressure on a study to produce an authoritative answer. Unfortunately, studies performed in the field of nutritional treatments over several decades may be perceived as being unhelpful for this reason, because they are complex and the conclusions are not always clear or easy to understand. To those not involved in research, it might appear that the conclusion from an RCT, even a negative or equivocal one, is the only type of conclusion that they can depend on. However, as with many important aspects of our lives, it's the details of these nutritional studies that are vital. It's important to understand as many of the details as possible and to have a positive outlook, because millions of people are using vitamin supplements to help prevent eye disease. Although some studies have not shown a benefit,[86] the outlook for preventing eye disease with nutrition has gotten better as more knowledge is accumulated.

Many of the classic orthomolecular treatments, for example, vitamin C given at high doses to treat viral infections, or vitamins C and E to treat heart disease, were discovered by pioneering doctors who tried to find the best treatment, then developed and tested hypotheses and published the results from their own clinical records.[87] This type of observational evidence, although very meaningful and important, may be ignored by scientists unfamiliar with the mechanisms likely responsible for it. For those not familiar with the background observational evidence, useful hypotheses that can be correctly tested with an RCT may be difficult to develop. Indeed, the strong results from clinical studies of orthomolecular treatment are often dismissed as originating in patient or doctor bias, for example, incorrectly diagnosing a patient's symptoms. Orthomolecular medicine would be more widely understood and accepted if strong positive results about the nutritional approach could be derived from RCTs. For example, when a clinical test of different doses of a nutrient provides data on the efficacy of these different doses (the proportionality paradigm above), this can suggest doses for testing by RCTs. Although there have been several recent observational studies showing that high doses of vitamin D can prevent or reverse flu and multiple sclerosis,[88] and reduce risk of macular degeneration,[89] it is rare to see an RCT employ high doses of vitamin C, vitamin E, or any of a dozen other orthomolecular treatments. In fact, there have been very few RCTs done to test a scientific question about orthomolecular nutrition with the proper doses. This may be because nutrition is very complex and depends on many factors, including genetic makeup, interactions between foods and nutrients, and differences in the daily diet and stress levels. Simple scientific questions such as the effect of a low dose of one nutrient do not always give clear answers. Thus, the overall approach of orthomolecular medicine is to search, given what we know about the effect of nutrition on the body, for the most effective combinations of nutrients in an excellent diet.

PUBLIC ACCESS TO SCIENCE

To grasp the critical issues involved in health studies about vitamin supplements, it is important to have access to the background knowledge that enables one to understand the known causes of disease and the rationale behind treating with supplements. Historically this knowledge was contained in the scientific literature as articles in scientific journals, which are critically peer-reviewed and thus have, at least, been accepted and verified by a group of experts. To learn about a health topic such as macular degeneration, one can go to a university library and look up review articles, which contain references to a variety of other basic findings. One could read the articles in the library and take notes, or in recent decades, one could photocopy the articles to read later.

Another way to learn about body function and health is to buy or borrow a book. Many health books are available, and some are extremely useful for quickly grasping a topic such as nutrients and health. The most useful ones give a clear description of the basic facts and issues and lots of references. Then, to make the best use of the book, one should check the references. In the past, this path led back to the library, where one could look up the articles and read them. This is always a good way to learn about a topic.

However, in the last several decades several important developments have taken place in access to medical knowledge. One of them is the availability of online encyclopedias, Weblogs, and wikis. These allow anyone with Internet access to read the facts and hypotheses about almost any topic, including the body organs, diseases, nutrients, and the benefit of supplements. This has brought about a revolution in access to knowledge. However, to utilize these wikis most efficiently, one soon learns some informal but very important rules. Online blogs and wikis are subject to continual updates, so their content may change over a period of days, leading the casual reader to wonder whether their content is trustworthy. It becomes obvious that to trust what one reads, one needs a way to verify.

The most basic rule continues to be "Check the references." In science, every hypothesis and conclusion must be backed up by references, and publications that review a topic, attempting to state current knowledge, are completely dependent on their reference section. If someone writes a scientific review-for example, the recent review article about macular degeneration by de Jong,[90] that is chockfull of references—the review's contents are authoritative and completely accurate. But upon reading such an article lacking plentiful references, the reader would not be able to verify the accuracy. This ability to verify statements is the critical factor that gives assurance that the facts presented are correct and that the hypotheses are reasonable. For this reason, online articles of blogs and wikis that are well-documented with references can be very powerful. Even though the opinions expressed will invariably reflect the personal bias of their authors, the careful reader will take this into account when checking the references. This is also the reason that articles or books without any references, although they may be completely correct, are generally not as useful for learning and verifying knowledge. The same is true for the Internet. The best online blogs and wikis are those that provide adequate references.

Another important development in health knowledge is PubMed, the official site of the National Institutes of Health for searching the literature. While PubMed does not index all medical literature, it does index a large fraction, allowing anyone with Internet access to look up articles in a variety of ways, for example, by author, topic, journal, or year. This is very relevant to the topic of vitamins and their health benefits, because much of the recent flurry of research on vitamins is available online. When you enter one or more search criteria (typically an author's name and/or a topic) and click on the "search" button, the PubMed site responds with a list of article titles that meet the search criteria. You can then click on the titles to get more information about them.

Many articles contain an abstract on their first page. This is a summary of the article's purpose, methods, results, and conclusions, often limited in length to perhaps 250 words. If it is a review article it will summarize knowledge from other papers, but it may describe methods and results from those papers, as well as background information from the cited papers, and their conclusions. All of these may be summarized in the abstract. In PubMed the abstracts are often presented, free to the public, when they are available. This is helpful because it allows you to quickly ferret out basic ideas. Browsing quickly through abstracts in PubMed can allow you to locate literature that you are interested in without getting bogged down in details. However, when the main text of many papers is not freely available, it is quite common for researchers to read abstracts without critically evaluating and verifying the conclusions. This is unfortunate, because reading abstracts cannot substitute for careful reading of the complete manuscripts and their references.

Because references are so important, they can be a good way to expand your knowledge about a topic On first reading, you may not understand all of the words and ideas in a review article. But by checking the references and reading the relevant background articles, you can eventually discover all the background you need. When necessary you can in turn check the reference section of the background articles, reading these older papers to construct a tree of knowledge based on published references. This is one way that scientists develop background knowledge. However, this method of finding references can only go backwards in time. If the original review article was published many years ago, it obviously cannot refer to recent developments in the same topic. To circumvent this problem, you can use a citation index. Typically you look up a classic article that you know was important in a field, usually by the author's name and year. The citation index lists the (more recent) papers that refer to this older classic paper. In this way, you can find more recent articles on the same or similar topic. If some of these more recent articles are review papers, this gives you a handle to quickly expand your search to find lot: of other relevant recent papers. The citation indexes are typically not available free to the public, but many university libraries subscribe to them.

Another important recent development in access to health knowledge is PubMed Central, which is a database of biomedical and life sciences containing the complete full-length articles, freely available to the public. It was initiated by the United States Congress when it passed a bill specifying that all research funded by the National Institutes of Health, from the year 2008 onward, should be made freely available. The law allows scientific journals to delay availability of this free version by up to one year so they can recoup the cost of the articles through subscriptions. Many journals allow papers from previous years to be republished by PubMed Central, which has become an excellent free online archive of biomedical research. You can find these free articles by a search in PubMed. When you click on the title to see the abstract, an icon may appear saying "Freely Available in PubMed Central." Click on this icon and you'll get a link to the free public version of the article.

A final word of caution: If you find health-related Web sites or printed pamphlets, published by private institutions or associated with the government, that caution about the effectiveness of vitamin supplements, try to understand the rationale for the advice. Are references provided, and if you read the references, can you understand them? Very often, health Web sites give a variety of advisory statements, explaining that there is "little evidence" for the action of a supplement, for example, vitamin C. Many such sites continue to give conservative advice that is out of date and misleading. Such advice is not necessarily disingenuous or incorrect, as it may be based on valid research that is applicable to some people. But remember from the paragraphs above that any health study must address a specific scientific question. If the scientific question is limited in scope and the study does not find a convincing answer, it does not obviate the value of older or more recent evidence that, for example, vitamin C at high doses is very helpful and safe. Science continues to progress, and the advisories must be continually updated. To check such advisories, find the most relevant section of this book and look up the references to see how they compare.

CHAPTER 3

THE EYE: HOW IT WORKS, AND WHAT CAN GO WRONG

The eye is an exquisite organ, marvelous because it gives us sight but also because of its intricate structure.[91] The eye is tough and resilient enough to last for a lifetime but is also very delicate. Its nearly spherical shape is crucial for its proper function to rotate and view the world and to control and focus light rays. This special shape is maintained by a slightly elevated internal pressure, which makes it susceptible to pressure-related problems.

STRUCTURE OF THE EYE

The eye is rotated by six muscles attached from the side of the eyeball to the back of the orbit in the skull. The front of the eye is protected by a transparent lining called the cornea, which is lubricated and nourished externally by tears and internally by a fluid inside the eye called the aqueous humor (see Figure 3.1).

The lubrication of the cornea by tears allows our eyelids to move up and down. It is a delicate tissue that can easily be damaged. Inside the eye, behind the cornea and aqueous humor, sits the iris, which regulates the amount of light that can pass into the back of the eye. It opens and closes the pupil like the diaphragm of a camera lens. Just behind the iris sits the lens, which has a high refractive index and bends light rays to focus an image of the world on the back of the eye. The high refractive index of the lens is due to a clear crystalline protein contained in its cells. Around its edge, the lens is attached to muscles in the ciliary body that control where the eye is focused. Behind the lens, a gel-like transparent liquid called the vitreous humor fills most of the eye. It can contain particles and detritus from the eye tissues that cause "floaters" in our vision.

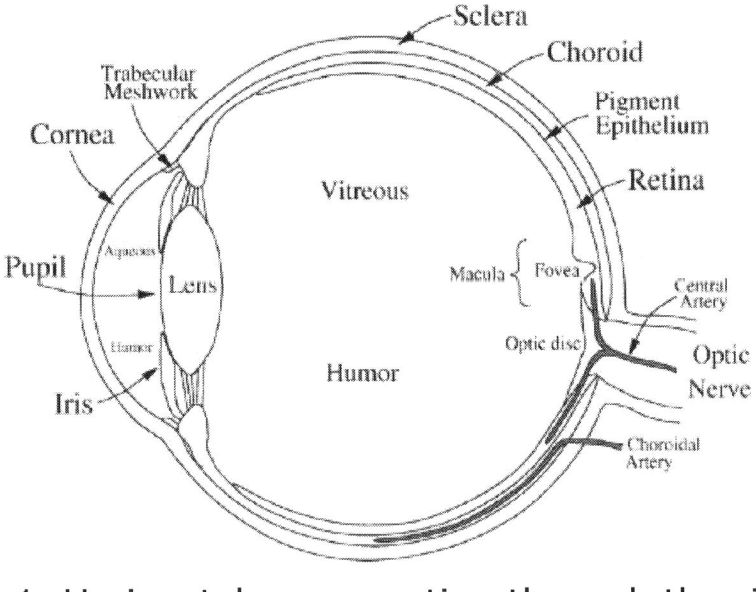

Figure 3.1. Horizontal cross-section through the right eye, showing its basic structure. Intraocular pressure on the sclera sets the eye's spherical shape. At the front of the eye, the cornea, pupil, and lens transmit light which passes through the vitreous to the retina at the back of the eye. The retina is held in place by the pigment epithelium, the inner lining of the choroid, which contains blood vessels that nourish the pigment epithelium and retina. Retinal blood vessels originate from the ophthalmic artery.

Ganglion cells on the inner surface of the retina send their axons to the optic disk where they form the optic nerve. (Adapted with permission from Smith, R.G. "Nutrition and eye disease." J Orthomol Med 25(3rd Quarter), 2010.)

The Retina

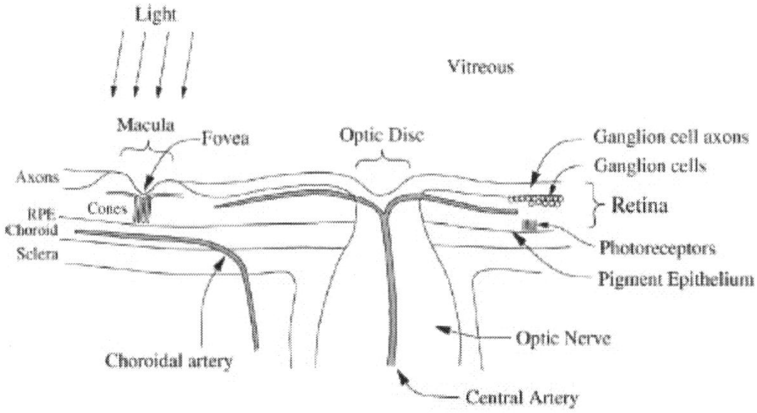

Figure 3.2. Horizontal section through the back of the left eye from above, showing the optic disk where the optic nerve emanates from the eye. Light passes through the lens and vitreous, through the retina, and is absorbed by the photoreceptors (rods, cones). The fovea, which provides higher solution vision, consists entirely of cones, which must send their signals laterally to connect to the second-order neurons. The macula is the region extending from the fovea outwards several degrees, containing an orange-y yellowish pigment that protects the pho-toreceptors. The retinal pigment epithelium (RPE) is a thin layer of cells that nurture and regenerate the photoreceptor outer segments. The choroid, below the RPE, supplies nutrients to the pigment epithelial cells and the photoreceptors. Ganglion cells at the surface send their axons along the retinal surface, converging at the optic nerve. The retina is supplied with blood from the ophthalmic artery that sends a fine branch as the central artery in the optic nerve, which is paired with a central vein (not illustrated). The choroid is supplied by a separate plexus of

arteries. The sclera is a tough outer membrane that contains the eye's pressure and holds its spherical shape.

Near the back of the eye, attached to the eyeball's inner lining, sits the retina. This is where the process of vision starts. At the back of the retina, a layer of cells called photoreceptors convert the light into electrical impulses, which are coded by three layers of cells into visual signals. These cells are types of "neurons;" which means they are like all the other cells in the body except they have special properties. Neurons are electrically excitable, and they can pass electrical information on to their neighbors at sites called "synapses;" by releasing tiny packets of chemicals called neurotransmitters.[92] These visual signals are carried by the axons of ganglion cells across the surface of the retina to the optic disk, where they exit the eyeball and become the optic nerve that carries visual impulses to the brain (Figure 3.2).

The optic disk is also called the "blind spot," because at this location the retina contains no photoreceptors. You can find your blind spot by making two small spots about five inches apart on a piece of paper. Hold the piece of paper with the spots along a horizontal line, close one eye, and look at the spot closest to your nose, (for your right eye, look at the left spot). Move the paper closer and farther away, ten to fifteen inches from your eyes, while continuing to fixate on the spot, and at some point the other spot will disappear. That is your blind spot, and it is completely normal. For most of our lives we never notice this small spot of blindness, for the brain makes up (confabulates) a consistent visual scene that obscures this spot. Our vision is surprisingly wide, up to 180 degrees horizontally and up to 100 degrees vertically. You can look for other blind spots or "sco-tomas" by wiggling your fingers while moving your hand around each eye's visual space, especially in the periphery. This type of testing is performed by medical professionals to map damage to the retina and visual part of the brain.

The photoreceptors consist of cones and rods, which differ in their sensitivity to light (Figure 3.3, opposite). Cones in apes and humans come in three types, with different visual pigments that absorb the three primary colors. Many other species, such as fish, turtles, and birds, have excellent color vision, but most mammalian species have only two cone types and therefore a limited ability to see color. Cones only respond to bright light, for example, from dawn to dusk. Rods come in only one variety and they are exquisitely sensitive, able to respond to a single photon.[93] They are much more numerous than cones—90 million rods vs 4.5 million cones[94]—and are most active in the dark of night, so they are responsible for most of the energy use of the retina. Both rods and cones can readily adapt to different light levels. The retina is attached to a layer of cells called the retinal pigment epithelium (RPE), that nourish and care for the outer segments of the photoreceptors.[95] Behind the RPE sits the choroid, a matrix of blood vessels supplying nourishment to the pigment epithelium and retina. The retina is also supplied with oxygen and nutrients from an internal network of blood vessels that are arranged in two layers. They are supplied by a branch of the ophthalmic artery that courses through the center of the optic nerve (Figure 3.2).

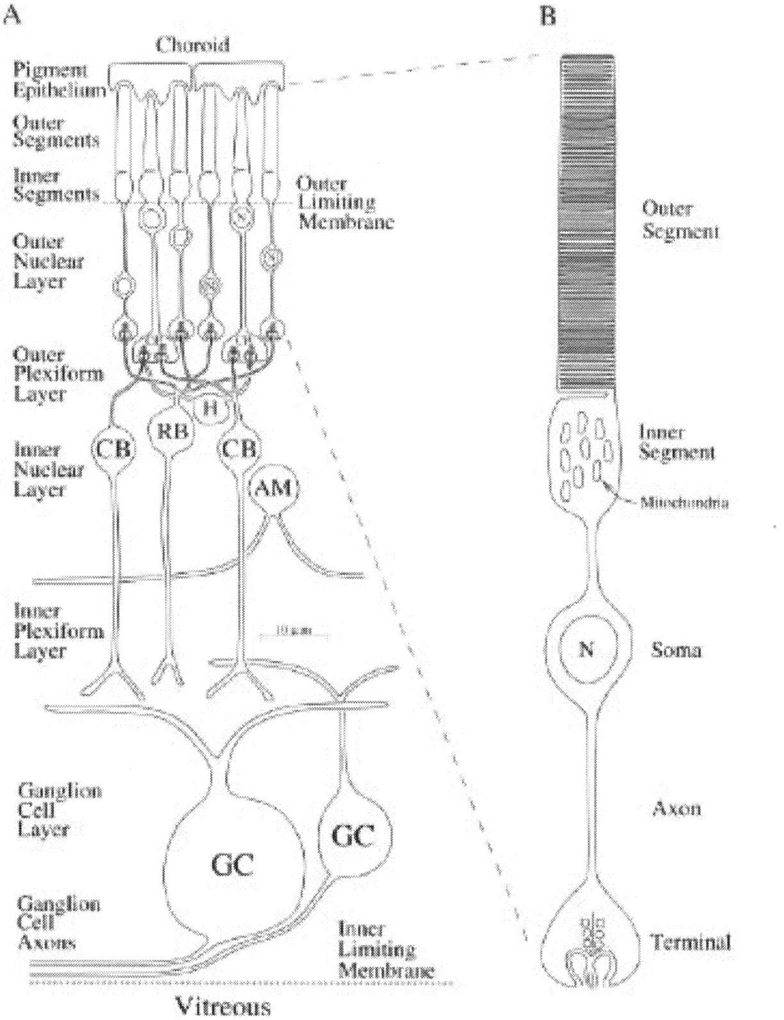

Figure 3.3. Organization of the Retina. A. The photoreceptor layer consists of rods and cones. Their outer segments interface with the pigment epithelium. Photoreceptors make synaptic connections to bipolar cells and horizontal cells (H). Bipolar cells carry the visual signal from the outer to the inner retina. Rod bipolar cells (RB) carry rod signals and are active at night. Cone bipolar cells (CB) carry cone signals, responsible for color vision, and are active in the day. Amacrine cells (AM) make synaptic connections with bipolar cells and ganglion cells (GC) and perform spatial and temporal processing. Bipolar cells make synaptic connections to ganglion cells, which send the visual signal through

their axons to the brain. (For more details on retinal circuitry, see R.W. Rodieck, The First Steps in Seeing, 1998.) B. Higher magnification image of a rod photoreceptor, showing the outer and inner segments, soma with nucleus (N), axon, and terminal containing its output synapse. The outer segment comprises several hundred discs that contain rhodopsin, the visual pigment. The discs are made of lipid membrane, containing a large fraction of poly unsaturated omega-3 fatty acids, which are prone to oxidative damage from toxins, oxy gen, and light. The outer segment discs of photoreceptors contain more membrane lipids than other retinal cell types, so they are the most susceptible to this type of oxidative stress.

Near the center of the retina sits a region called the "fovea:" This is a special region of the retina that contains only cone photoreceptors, which are responsible for our ability to see color in daylight (Figure 3.2). We utilize the fovea to see fine details and to read. It is about two degrees in diameter, with cones crammed into a regular triangular packing. To give the cones a better chance of absorbing light, and to prevent distortion and diffraction by other neurons, the fovea excludes all other types of neurons, including rod photoreceptors. The foveal cones send their axons (the "fibers of Henle") laterally to contact the second-order neurons. In this para-foveal region (2–10 degrees from the center of the retina), called the macula, some rods are mixed in with the cones. The macular region has no blood vessels within the retina, and is supplied with nutrients and oxygen by blood vessels in the choroid, beneath the RPE. Thus the macula is especially susceptible to hypoxia (low level of oxygen). Farther from the fovea, in the peripheral retina, the cones gradually get farther apart, until they are each surrounded by hundreds of rods. The overall organization of the rods and cones gives us the highest resolution possible in the fovea and the most efficient absorption of photons at night by rods in the periphery. This is the reason we are blind in our central vision at night—there are no rods in the fovea. It is also the reason that we don't have good visual acuity in our peripheral vision. If you try to read a newspaper, even its headline, you will find it impossible when you're not directly looking at it with your fovea. To see a faint star at night, you must look away from it to allow your rods to capture its photons. But you can see planets and bright stars in the same nighttime sky by looking directly at them, using your foveal cones.

The retina and all other parts of the brain and spinal cord are within the "blood-brain barrier," which protects the brain from outside influences such as bacteria, viruses, toxins, and many drugs. On the inside wall of each blood vessel, endothelial cells sit ready to protect the brain. They are connected with a system of tight junctions so that their cell membranes are very closely apposed, which prevents large molecules or anything else larger, such as viruses, from getting through. Even glucose is too big to get through the tight junctions. Glucose and all other essential biochemicals the brain needs are transported through the endothelial cells by special protein transporters in their membranes.[96] All blood vessels, even the microscopically fine (seven-micron diameter) capillaries, are protected by the blood-brain barrier. It is as if a complete firewall is protecting your brain from chemicals and viruses emanating from the environment. When this blood-retinal barrier becomes dysfunctional, neurological disease quickly results.

The blood-brain barrier has several consequences for the retina. First, the blood vessels of the retina must be quite tough to resist attack by viruses, bacteria, and antibodies, yet they must be thin and transparent to light. Second, nutrient molecules that the retina needs must all be recognized and transported through the blood-brain barrier by the endothelial cells, but the rate of transport is limited by the endothelial cells' natural abilities. Third, any chemicals or drugs that are not essential nutrients may have a difficult time getting into the retina or any other part of the brain.[97] This is one reason why acute diseases of the retina may be difficult to treat with drugs, or even with big doses of vitamin supplements—the retina is largely protected from outside influence. But in some cases, chemicals that have the same 3D configuration as essential nutrients can be transported through the blood-brain barrier, as can lipophilic chemicals, such as vitamin E, that naturally diffuse into cell membranes.

The eye contains many conundrums, and to unravel them takes knowledge and intuition about its delicate structure and necessary function. For example, on first thought, the retina may seem to be inside out. The ganglion cells are on the surface, adjacent to the vitreous humor, where they are first exposed to light passing into the eye. The photoreceptors are underneath, at the back of the retina. Light must pass through the entire depth of the retina, through its three layers of neurons, before the photoreceptors get a chance to absorb it. Why is the retina constructed this way? Why not have the ganglion cells underneath and the photoreceptor cells on the surface, where they would intercept the incoming light without any interference? The reason, of course, is unknown—all we can say for sure is what happens and how. But speculating on this type of conundrum can help us gain insight.

Although the retina is very thin, only 100–200 microns thick (about 1/10 millimeter [mm]), its supply of sugar (glucose) and oxygen is critical for its survival. The problem is that the neurons of the retina, and especially the photoreceptors, need a lot of sugar (glucose) and oxygen because their metabolic rate is one of the highest in the body. If the photoreceptors were on the surface of the retina, they would require a matrix of blood vessels close by to get enough nutrition, for this is evidently the purpose of the mat of blood vessels that make up the choroid. If the blood vessels were on the surface of the retina they would absorb and diffract light meant for the photoreceptors, preventing clear vision. Further, to keep the photoreceptors ready to absorb and transduce photons into electrical signals, they require the RPE cells to regenerate the pigment molecules and digest and recycle the old used discs of membrane into their component bio-chemicals. And further, the RPE cells in many species contain a layer of reflective pigment called the tapetum that acts like a mirror to give any photons not initially absorbed by the outer segments of the photoreceptor a second chance to be seen. Apparently the retina's high metabolic rate and its need for helper RPE cells to digest and reflect are the reason for the retina's complex inside out structure. Although the structure may seem nonintuitive at first, it has been designed by evolution as a compromise to give maximal performance.

The retina is a three-layered structure that looks from a distance like a piece of wet tissue paper—and is almost as delicate. It is held to the back of the eye by the RPE cells that contact and care for the photoreceptors. One problem with this arrangement is that the retina is easily separated from the RPE by a physical shock like a hard blow or by a pressure change that affects the eyeball's shape. Another problem is that the photoreceptors are severely stressed by bright light, which causes a variety of symptoms including deposits of oxidized biochemicals. These oxidized deposits can build up over many years, causing retinal detachment or other problems that can lead to blindness.

Eye doctors are trained to diagnose dozens of different diseases from a simple eye exam, and for some diseases they can prescribe a drug treatment that will help to ameliorate the symptoms. However, many eye diseases are thought to be incurable because no drug will prevent or reverse them. The tragedy of age-related eye disease is that, although some of its specific causes such as genetic factors and aging are being worked out (albeit at a very slow pace), many people, including medical professionals, are unaware of the abundant evidence linking optimum nutrition to eye-disease prevention and reversal.

OXIDATIVE STRESS AND ANTIOXIDANTS

The biological machinery of life can be damaged in many ways, and the eye is especially susceptible because it is a delicate organ on the body's surface. Although oxygen is used to metabolize food efficiently and thus provide energy, it also can cause damage. An oxygen molecule readily binds to many biochemicals by pulling electrons from them, which damages them. This can result in molecules with a free unbound and energized electron, known as "free radicals;" which are highly reactive.[98] When many molecules in a tissue are damaged in this way, the tissue has "oxidative stress." The free radicals then damage other biomolecules by pulling away electrons, generating more free radicals. These generate others, and so on, so that many molecules are damaged in sequence. This can wreak havoc with the machinery of life inside each cell. The cell membrane, its enzymes, and its DNA can all be damaged by oxidative stress. If enough damage occurs, the cell may die, or even worse, be transformed into a cancer cell that starts to grow without limit.

Oxidative stress can also be caused by many different types of damage to the eye, including physical damage (cuts or bruises), viral or bacterial infections, chemical toxins such as smoke, oxidative ions such as iron, and free radicals generated by light. A photon can get absorbed by a biomolecule, which may cause the molecule to generate a free radical, similar to what happens in a reaction with oxygen. Therefore, the eye is particularly at risk. It is designed to receive and absorb light, but light inherently causes an oxidizing reaction. Chemical toxins in the environment, such as smoke, are also easily able to induce oxidative stress. Smoke contains literally several thousand highly toxic chemicals, many of which are free radicals that are carcinogenic and can directly cause oxidative damage.[99] And a virus carried by a microscopic drop of water may land on the eye, causing an infection followed by inflammation and oxidative stress. Thus, the eye needs protection from oxidative stress due to environmental toxins, iron, and light.

To put these facts in perspective, it is also known that oxidative stress is a normal cellular response to environmental stimuli such as physical damage and exposure to toxins. Cells depend to some extent on oxidized molecules for signaling within the cell, and may require some oxidative stress to accelerate the production of internal antioidants, biochemical pathways responsible for tissue repair, and response to exercise.[100] Thus, the goal of dietary supplementation with antioxidants is not to completely remove oxidative stress everywhere throughout the body. Rather, the role of dietary antioxidants is to support the body's natural defenses and repair mechanisms. This underscores the orthomolecular approach to dietary supplementation with natural biomolecules essential for the body. A natural molecule such as vitamin C or vitamin E is less likely than artificial antioxidants or drugs to cause disruption of essential signaling pathways within cells and tissues. Because most animals make large amounts of vitamin C (equivalent to 10,000mg daily for adult humans), and this dose has been tested many times in studies, it is thought to be appropriate, helpful, and safe.

Oxidative Stress and Eye Disease

The eye defends against oxidative stress with antioxidants such as vitamin C, vitamin E, and glutathione.[101] Because it is small and highly mobile, vitamin C will react quickly with a free radical, donating an electron, which "reduces" the free radical and removes its reactivity. The vitamin C molecule, in turn, gets oxidized by the removal of two electrons. Its oxidized form, dehydroascorbic acid (DHAA), can be recycled into the active reduced form by red blood cells. Because it is water soluble, vitamin C is readily excreted by the kidneys—but not before it does its job of helping to prevent oxidative stress. Vitamin C is carried throughout the body in the bloodstream and gets transported into cells where it immediately goes to work, helping to maintain a reducing environment inside the cell. A cell containing sufficient vitamin C can prevent free radicals diffusing through its cytoplasm from damaging its DNA and intricate metabolic pathways. Because the eye has an unusually high level of oxidative stress, it concentrates vitamin C in the aqueous by a factor of twenty-five (to 1.1

millimolar) over the blood serum level. This high level of vitamin C is thought to directly obviate oxidative damage caused by light.[102]

Vitamin C can also regenerate other antioxidants such as vitamin E and glutathione when their active reducing form gets depleted by their function to combat oxidative stress.[103] Because vitamin E is fat soluble (lipophilic), it normally sits in the lipid bilayer of the cell's membrane where it prevents oxidation of the fatty acids and proteins that make up the membrane. Vitamin E is often added to polyunsaturated oils to prevent them from going rancid (oxidized). Without sufficient antioxidant capacity, many highly nutritious oil-containing foods such as wheat germ will go rancid in a few weeks when stored at room temperature. The same basic reaction happens inside the body, but it is controlled by antioxidants. Some of these, such as glutathione, can be generated afresh by the body, but others such as vitamin E must come from the diet. The body, using special-purpose enzymes to facilitate the reaction, can regenerate most antioxidants back into their reduced form. The enzymes are important because the antioxidants are crucial. Glutathione is so ubiquitous in the body that the ratio of oxidized to reduced glutathione is often used as a measure of the amount of oxidative stress. Thus, antioxidants are essential to keep our cells functioning normally and prevent mutations in a cell's DNA. They are crucial for all life, from bacteria to plants to animals.[104]

Beyond its role as an antioxidant, vitamin C is also essential for the synthesis of collagen, the most common protein in the body and a crucial component of the body's organs, blood vessels, and skin. Other antioxidants may also have additional functions, for example, some recent evidence suggests that vitamin E may also act in other ways as a messenger inside cells to help reduce damage.[105] Vitamin B_2(riboflavin), important for the metabolism of the body, is also an antioxidant. Lutein and zeaxanthin are important antioxidants found in the eye, but they double as filters of blue light.

Many lines of evidence imply that oxidative stress is a major factor in age-related eye diseases.[106] Early studies showed that aging eyes received an immediate benefit in vision from 600 milligrams (mg) per day of supplemental vitamin C. The benefit appeared throughout the retina, optic nerve, and the eye's vasculature,[107] and existed for patients who did not have an acute vitamin-C deficiency. The eye can also easily be damaged by free radicals in the bloodstream that are caused by environmental toxins like smoke and pesticides. Smokers have lower vitamin C levels in the bloodstream, throughout the body, and especially in the eye, so they are at risk for age-related eye diseases. Obesity is also a risk factor for eye disease. The cause is apparently an increased oxidation of lipids and a lower production of antioxidant compounds such as glutathione.[108] Diabetes is also a risk factor for eye disease, because high levels of blood sugar increase oxidative stress.[109] When eye tissues are damaged by oxidative stress, they require more energy to maintain life because their metabolism does not function as efficiently. They become stressed by any lack of nutrients essential for metabolic reactions.[110]

You may already know that green leafy vegetables are good for your health. Surprisingly, the carotenoids lutein and zeaxanthin, the principal carotenoid pigments in corn, peppers, and green leafy vegetables, are the primary constituents of the macular filter that removes blue light on the path to the retina. They are also found inside the outer segments of photoreceptors, where the concentration of omega-3 polyunsaturated fatty acids is the highest, and therefore is where the eye is most susceptible to oxidative damange. Lutein is a powerful antioxidant, because it can quench singlet oxygen radicals and then return to its original state by dissipating heat.[111] Thus for this reaction lutein is more useful than vitamin E, which requires regeneration by another antioxidant such as vitamin C. Lutein also has potent anti-inflammatory effects, and is thought to assist in repairing breaks in DNA from light exposure that contribute to cell death.[112] Lutein and zeaxanthine are "low oxygen" antioxidants, and are found in the inner retina where there is less oxygen. They are also found in other structures throughout the eye and therefore are essential to the health of the retina. They are thought to lessen oxidative stress throughout the retina, but especially in the macula, the retina's central region. A diet supplemented with lutein and zeaxanthin thus lowers the risk for eye disease.[113] Although lutein and zeaxanthin are almost identical, varying in the direction of only one chemical bond, they differ in their distribution in the retina. Zeaxanthin is found mainly in the macula, and lutein is found mainly in the periphery of the eye.[114] Vitamin E is a "high oxygen" antioxidant. It is relatively more efficient at removing oxidative stress in the outer retina, where there is more oxygen.[115] Vitamin E is helpful in preventing oxidative stress to photoreceptors[116] but it can also help to lower intraocular pressure. Further, antioxidants such as vitamin E and glutathione have synergistic effects.[117]

These lines of evidence are all related, because oxidative stress spreads relatively indiscriminately throughout cells and tissue, and any antioxidant will help prevent it. Vitamin E, which is fat soluble, sits in cell membranes and can quench free radicals in membrane lipids (fats) and proteins, but to be useful after this protective action, it must be reduced again. This can be accomplished by a water-soluble antioxidant such as vitamin C.[118] Natural antioxidants concentrated in mitochondria are thought to be essential for preventing oxidative damage.[119] New "designer" antioxidants, constructed with properties that target mitochondria, have been found to prevent damage in RPE cells, extend the life of laboratory mice, and prevent oxidative eye damage in dogs, cats, and horses.[120] Thus, a variety of different lines of evidence imply that antioxidants are important in preventing oxidative damage in the eye. It only makes sense, then, that eye diseases that typically progress with age are caused at least in part by oxidative damage that builds up when there is an insufficient level of antioxidants available to counteract it.

CHAPTER 4

THE EFFECTS OF LIGHT ON THE EYE

The eye is the only part of the body besides the skin, nails, and hair that is exposed to strong T ultraviolet (UV) and blue light for long periods. Light rays can damage the eye when they pass through its internal structures such as the lens and retina. When these structures absorb some of the light passing through them, it can oxidize the bio-chemicals and generate free radicals that further damage the essential proteins and DNA throughout the eye.[121] The transparent tissues of the eye, including the cornea, lens, vitreous, and retina, all absorb a small fraction of the light they transmit, and thus are susceptible to oxidative damage. If you go outside on a bright, sunny day, your eyes may absorb 100 trillion (1014) photons per second, which they can deal with for a few hours. The damage is small and the eye repairs itself, but nevertheless some permanent damage remains. Although each eye structure passes more than 90 percent of the light it receives, overall only about 50 percent of the light reaches the photoreceptors at the back of the retina. Over many years of exposure, for example three decades (10,950 days), repeated exposure to bright light causes an accumulation of damage that the eye cannot repair. This is why advice to wear dark glasses and wide-brimmed hats outside is well heeded. You can minimize your eyes' exposure to oxidative stress by avoiding long exposure to sources of bright light, such as the blue sky.

NEED AND RISK OF UV LIGHT EXPOSURE

Ironically, we need exposure to short-wavelength UV light, called UVB, to synthesize vitamin D in our skin. Long-wavelength UV light, or UVA, is the stimulus that causes our skin to darken or tan. UVA is more prevalent because less is absorbed by the atmosphere, but we only need a small amount of exposure to UVB to get enough vitamin D. It is important to remember that going outside in the sunlight has a benefit. To get an adequate amount of vitamin D, you need ten minutes of exposure daily to the midday summer sun on your back, legs, and arms if you have light skin.[122] If you have dark skin you may need up to an hour of sun exposure daily, or several hours of exposure to your arms and legs. Remember that during this time you should limit your eye exposure to bright light. The easiest way, as mentioned above, is to put on a wide-brimmed hat and dark glasses, preferably a pair that filters out blue and UV light.

Vitamin D has many beneficial effects for the body, including the regulation of calcium in the tissues and bones, prevention of many types of cancer, and prevention of macular degeneration (see Macular Degeneration). But getting vitamin D through exposure to sunlight can be a two-edged sword, because in addition to its long-term effects on the eye, exposure to bright light can cause skin cancer (melanoma) that is fast-growing and life-threatening. The worst offenders are blue light and UV because these have the highest energy per photon, and therefore they can do more damage when absorbed by a molecule. Exposure to winter sunlight for several hours in the northern states of the United States and Canada can give you a tan, but provides hardly any vitamin D. For this reason exposure to bright winter sunlight should be avoided to prevent eye damage. So the best advice is, during the summer, expose your skin but not your eyes to midday sunlight for a few minutes when possible, but otherwise minimize your exposure to bright light, especially direct sunlight. To know whether you are getting enough vitamin D, you should take a blood test for the level of 25-hydroxyvitamin D. The blood test is readily available at most clinics, and considering its benefits, it is relatively inexpensive. If you are low in vitamin D, you should take vitamin D supplements (35–50 international units [IU] per pound of body weight per day, or for average adults, 5,00010,000IU per day) for several months and then get tested again. The reason for this is that vitamin D, being a fat-soluble vitamin, builds up slowly in the body.

Most of the UV light passing into the eye is absorbed by the cornea and lens,[123] but much of the blue light is transmitted to the retina, which has one of the highest metabolic rates of any tissue in the body. Because the retina has near-arterial oxygen levels, higher than most other tissues, it has one of the highest risks of oxidative damage.[124] Further, it contains a high proportion of polyunsaturated fatty acids, located in the bilayered structure of cell membranes, that can be easily damaged by oxidation.[125] Mitochondria, located in retinal neurons, are necessary for the retina's high metabolic rate. They are subcellular organelles, thought to have evolved from small bacteria-like cells that were absorbed by animal cells many millions of years ago. They are responsible for our ability to metabolize food to generate energy, and they contain cytochromes, which are biochemicals involved in energy metabolism that are colored due to their chemical structure. Cytochromes absorb light because of their color, and this process can generate free radicals, damaging the cell's metabolism and also its ability to recover from further damage.[126] In addition, photoreceptors have an especially high polyunsaturated-fatty-acid content due to their disc structure. When a photon is absorbed by a polyunsaturated lipid, it can easily be damaged and generate a free radical.

The iris helps prevent the light damage by narrowing the aperture that allows light to pass into the eye. The pupil, the central open area in the iris that passes light, is controlled by the the brain according to the external light intensity. For protection against the effects of light, the iris contains a dark brown pigment, which is a melanin molecule similar to the pigment in skin, and this pigment absorbs light. Thus, people with blue eyes are at greater risk of damage because the blue color represents a lack of the light-absorbing pigment. If you habitually look at a bright TV or video screen in a dark room, or stare at the bright blue sky from inside a building, your iris may be dilated and the bright light may damage your eyes. Likewise, if you go out in the snow or a beach in the bright sunlight, over a period of years your eyes may be damaged by the extreme brightness of the scene. A good preventive measure is turn down the contrast on the video screen, and provide enough background light in the room to maintain a level of illumination about the same as the screen. Then your eye will properly adapt to the light level. If you're outside on bright days wear a wide-brimmed hat and dark glasses with yellowish lenses.

NORMAL AND PATHOLOGICAL FUNCTION OF LIGHT

The eye can recover and regenerate naturally from the many of the chemical reactions caused by light, as long as it isn't too intense. Photoreceptor pigment, opsin, is located in thin discs stacked in the outer segments of the photoreceptors at the back of the retina. Each molecule of opsin contains retinal, a submolecule that in the normal process of vision gets chemically modified (bleached) by absorbing a photon, and must be regenerated. The bleached retinal gets released from the opsin and is then transported into the retinal pigment epithelium (RPE) cells, which regenerate it and transport it back to the photoreceptors. In addition, the oldest discs are sloughed off at the outer tip of the outer segment to allow space for new discs to be created at the inner part of the outer segment. In a process called phagocytosis, the old discs at the photoreceptor tip are digested by the RPE.[127] New discs containing a fresh array of pigment molecules and enzymes are constructed at the base of the photoreceptor's outer segment, and over a period of days move progressively outward. Interestingly, whenever we are exposed to bright light such as sunlight, all of the pigment in our rod photoreceptors is bleached in a few minutes, which is the reason we get temporarily blinded when coming back inside to the dark interior of the house on a bright day. The pigment must be regenerated before we can see in the dark again, which takes forty-five to sixty minutes for full recovery.[128] The same thing happens from exposure to bright headlights when driving at night. We are partially blinded by even a short exposure to headlights and cannot see very well in the dark for at least fifteen minutes after this. The pigment is regenerated from vitamin A (retinyl or carotene), which as described above has been available in the diet of our ancestors for millions of years, so we must continue to obtain it from our food. This process is the normal working of vision, which the eye typically can keep up over our whole lifetime, as long as we keep eating enough carrots or dark green leafy vegetables.

But the tissues of the cornea, lens, and retina are damaged by photon absorption after years of exposure to bright light. Prolonged exposure to extremely bright light damages photoreceptors. The mechanism is not fully understood, but is thought to be related in part to a high level of bleaching of rhodopsin.[129] The damage is especially severe when a dark-adapted eye is exposed to bright light. When rod photoreceptors are exposed to varying levels of light, they get light-adapted, which reduces the amount of rhodopsin in their outer segments and prevents the damage.[130] Further, vitamin C is protective against the damage from bright light, but only when taken before the light exposure, implying that it directly prevents free-radical formation by light.[131] A further clue about this mechanism came from a study in which both the natural L-isomer of vitamin C and its D-stereoisomer were shown to be effective in preventing light dam-age.[132] Because both forms of vitamin C are known to be equally effective as antioxidants, but only the natural L-isomer is active in the other functions of vitamin C such as synthesis of collagen, this verified that the effect was due to the antioxidant function of vitamin C. A similar protective effect came from the L-isomer of N-acetyl-cysteine, a precursor of glutathione,[133] and also from many other antioxidant bioactive chemicals that quench hydrogen peroxide and hydroxyl radicals.[134]

Other molecules besides the opsin pigment can absorb photons but do not have the same regenerative capacity. A blue or UV photon has enough energy to break chemical bonds between atoms, and thus, when a photon is absorbed, it can generate a free radical that can attack nearby molecules. The synthesis of many types of proteins in retinal cells are affected by bright light, either due to direct oxidative damage or to compensatory regulation of their expression of necessary proteins.[135] Oxidative damage can build up and cause the eye's cells to stop functioning or die after many decades of exposure to sunlight. The damage happens quickly when the light is extremely bright, but builds up slowly over a lifetime with prolonged weaker exposure. These changes can be prevented by antioxidants, so it is important to take an adequate level of antioxidants such as vitamin C to prevent this type of damage to your eyes. According to the dynamic-flow model of vitamin-C utilization in the body, if you take vitamin C in divided doses throughout the day, for example 1–3 grams every four hours, you can maintain a high level throughout your body.[136]

Energy Use by Photoreceptors Exposed to Light

The vertebrate photoreceptor has a very high energy requirement, which impacts its ability to maintain its neural and cellular functions. In the dark, the energy use by rod and cone photoreceptors is maximal, because it is closely related to the ionic (electrical) current that flows into the outer segment.[137] To signal activation by light, the photoreceptors reduce the current flowing into the outer segment, which then reduces their release of neurotransmitter. In this way their metabolic energy pathways are less taxed when in light. This arrangement is specific to animals. In arthropods, such as insects, that have excellent vision, the photoreceptor cells use minimal energy in the dark and increase their electrical current in the light. On first thought, the arthropod mechanism for vision might appear to be more reasonable. The peculiar arrangement of the vertebrate photoreceptor's response to light and energy use begs the question why it functions this way. The facts about oxidative stress caused by light suggest the following hypothesis:

The photoreceptor requires energy to flow to its outer segment to deal with the normal bleaching of the visual pigment and oxidative stress caused by light. In the dark, when the photoreceptor's energy use is greater, it has little oxidative stress. In the light, when oxidative stress is greater, there is more energy available for the cell's metabolic pathways to support the light-driven signaling pathway in the outer segment.[138] However, this energy can also support the generation and transportation of other biochemicals necessary for maintenance, such as antioxidants. If the photoreceptors' response to light were to increase their use of energy, less energy would be available to fight the oxidative stress during the exposure to light. Thus the vertebrate photoreceptor's mechanism for signaling light allows it to devote more of its metabolic energy to fight oxidative stress. Although there may be additional reasons for this peculiar light signaling mechanism, this hypothesis seems appealing because it links the photoreceptor's metabolism with its need for maintenance.

Cataract: An Example of Oxidative Stress

A very common cause of vision loss after age sixty is cataract. This is a clouding of the lens in which the lens absorbs and scatters some of the light passing into the eye. The cloudy lens reduces the clarity of the image that the retina sees. Early in life, from young adulthood to middle age, the lens tissue is very transparent and actively repairs the lens proteins to keep itself intact. But with old age and the unavoidable damage due to oxidation from absorption of UV rays or ionizing radiation, the lens tissue cannot maintain itself in good condition.[139] Cataract is slow to develop and is not painful, so many people are not aware that their eyes have developed cataracts as they age. The problem is that the lens protein coagulates into small clumps, in a semicrystalline form, that look like tiny specks or spokes of a wheel. When this happens, absorbed water causes the lens to swell and it becomes cloudy. The standard treatment for cataract is surgery to remove the cloudy lens and replace it with a plastic insert. This surgery can be done safely on an outpatient basis in an ophthalmologist's office. The benefit is immediate, and many cataract patients can see well at different distances with proper glasses. It's easy to understand why this type of treatment is considered a miracle by those who've had their vision restored. However, many medical professionals are not aware of what can be done throughout adulthood to prevent the cataracts from forming in the first place.[140]

The basic causes of cataract are known. Oxidative stress causes the lens proteins to deteriorate, and this accelerates with age and exposure to light. People who live in sunny climates or spend a lot of time outside are at a higher risk for cataract. Airline pilots have a higher rate of cataract, thought to be caused by their exposure to oxidizing radiation from the upper atmosphere.[141] The atmosphere shields most of us from this damaging radiation, but there are other hazards. Genetic factors may increase the risk for cataract. People who smoke have a risk almost three times as great for cataract.[142] A likely reason is that smoking incurs an oxidative stress on the entire body, which greatly reduces the amount of vitamin C and vitamin E in the bloodstream.[143] Smokers tend to have higher levels of lead and cadmium in their blood and also in their eye lens, which is a risk factor for cataracts, because these toxic metal ions also tend to lower the level of vitamins C and E in the bloodstream.[144] Although there is no treatment to cure cataract currently, the onset can be delayed or prevented by an excellent diet with plenty of antioxidants.[145] Among the most important antioxidants useful in preventing cataract are lutein and zeaxanthin, which are the orange carotenoids present in dark green leafy vegetables.[146] The blood level of vitamin E is lower in patients with cataract, suggesting the use of vitamin E supplements to prevent cataract occurrence.[147] A supplement of vitamin C or vitamin E either alone, or combined with other antioxidants such as selenium and lipoic acid, is helpful in reducing the occurrence of cataracts.[148] This treatment is thought to remove free radicals and enhance the activity of glutathione in the eye, which is inversely related to the occurrence of cataract. Vitamin C has been shown to reduce the incidence of cataract if taken for at least a decade.[149]

Although antioxidants have been shown to be effective in preventing cataract in many observational studies, some randomized controlled trial (RCT) studies have found little or no effect. A recent study on the effect of vitamin C and vitamin E exemplifies this type of negative conclusion reached by some randomized controlled studies.[150] A large group of men (11,545), generally well-nourished, were given vitamin E or vitamin C over a period of several years. The study was designed to test the effect of these two important vitamins on the risk of cancer and cardiovascular disease, but the participants were also examined for cataracts, and their ophthalmologists were queried about the diagnosis and whether the cataracts had been removed by surgery. The conclusion, as stated in the summary of the study, was that long-term use of vitamin C or vitamin E had no effect, either beneficial or harmful, on the risk of cataract.[151]

However, a careful reading of the summary report reveals several important caveats. First, the levels of vitamin C and vitamin E were low by orthomolecular standards. Vitamin E was given at 400IU every other day. On first thought this might seem reasonable, because that dose is higher than typical dietary levels, and since vitamin E is fat soluble, it takes several weeks for its level to rise or fall in the body. However, a closer look reveals that the vitamin E used, dl-alpha-tocopherol, was the synthetic all-racemic form, and thus the effective dose was only half of the stated dose. The reason is that the naturally derived d-alpha-tocopherol form is preferentially taken up and utilized by the body, as are the other natural forms of vitamin E, d-beta, d-delta, and d-gamma, for both tocopherols and tocotrienols.[152]

The activity of the synthetic form of vitamin E, dl-alpha-tocopherol, can be measured in the test tube, but its biopotency in the body is only 50 percent of the natural form.[153] Taking these factors into account, the effective dose was only 100IU per day (one dose every other day, 50 percent bioavailability). Typical orthomolecular doses are in the range of 800–1,600IU per day, which is eight to sixteen times greater than the doses given in the study. The beneficial effect of nutrients such as vitamin E is known to be related to the dose, so it is apparent that the doses given were low by orthomolecular standards.[154]

Second, the participants were also randomly given daily beta-carotene and a daily multivitamin. However, no adjustment to the risk factors was made for the vitamin C and vitamin E in the multivitamin supplement, which contained 75 milligrams (mg) of vitamin C, and 70IU of vitamin E. Because of this, the randomized participants received a 70IU supplement of vitamin E, almost as much as the dose (effectively 100IU per day) that was being investigated. The effect of the multivitamin would be expected to confound any result from this study about vitamin E. If you are already taking some vitamin E, you can't expect a small additional amount to do much extra good for the body. And although a multivitamin supplement would be expected to provide an additional benefit due to the synergistic effect of its essential nutrients, this might be a small effect if the participants in the study were eating generous amounts of fresh vegetables and fruits, sprouts, whole grains, and yogurt.

Third, the dose of vitamin C given, 500mg per day, was also likely confounded by the vitamin C given in the multivitamin (75mg). This might not seem a problem, but it is known that the maintained level of vitamin C in the bloodstream from these relatively small single doses is similar,[155] and commonly those who are health-conscious will ingest 100–300mg from raw fruits and vegetables. To get a noticeable effect of an increased dose of vitamin C, you must take ten times this dose or more, for example, 5,000–10,000mg per day, taken in divided doses throughout the day. The divided doses (1,000–2,000mg) are well tolerated by most people, and when taken throughout the day they can increase the body's level of vitamin C several-fold.[156]

Fourth, although the study was conducted over eight to ten years, typically only a fraction of the participants fully complied over this period by taking all the pills. Compliance with the study was defined as those who had taken at least two thirds of the pills given to them, and there was only 78 percent compliance at four years. Cataract is thought to be related to oxidative stress over many decades, and thus common sense dictates that to prevent cataract, it will be necessary to eat a healthy diet with plenty of antioxidants over one's lifetime, starting as a young adult.

Additionally, any participants who were diagnosed with cataract at the start of the study were excluded, and those who developed cataract during the study were removed. This policy eliminated any possibility of discovering the potential effect of vitamin E for halting or reversal of cataract. Further, participants were also terminated from the study for reasons other than cataract. Because the study had originally been conducted to test the effect of supplements on the risk of cancer and heart disease, which are major debilitating diseases that may be related to risk factors for cataract, it appears likely that the results might have been biased by not taking into account those who got sick or died from these diseases. For example, those taking a placebo and thus not receiving the benefits of vitamin C or E may have had worse health, causing them to be more likely to develop heart disease. Those in the early stages of developing cataract would not be tabulated if they developed cancer or heart disease, which subsequently caused them to drop out of the study.

Finally, the study did show obvious beneficial effects for vitamin C and vitamin E for the younger participants (aged fifty to fifty-nine). The younger participants taking vitamin C had a 10 to 20 percent reduction in the risk for cataract, but this was not statistically significant as tabulated in the study, apparently because fewer younger participants were included. The younger participants taking vitamin E had a statistically significant 20 to 50 percent reduction (depending on the subgroup) in the risk for cataract if they took the relatively low dose specified. It seems possible that the older participants received less of an effect because cataract is relatively common and the rate increases with age. Given the study's provisions, the fraction of older people who tended to have cataracts would be eliminated from participating, leaving those who were in better health and thus not as likely to receive a benefit from the low levels of supplements given.

While there is a lot of detail to consider in such a study, an absence of a strong conclusion about vitamin supplements does not mean that they are not beneficial. It only means that with the doses given in the study, the effects of the treatments were not large enough to be obvious among random effects. Further, it doesn't mean that the study was designed or performed incorrectly. In this type of large expensive study, higher doses may have been avoided because of a preference to be conservative. While the official conclusion was "no effect;" it is easy to understand the lack of a strong conclusion given the study's problems. Moreover, when one looks closely at the results, the study did find a benefit for vitamin C and vitamin E in preventing cataract for middle-aged people, which is consistent with earlier observational studies.

Cataract can also be caused by high levels of blood sugar, a condition commonly found in diabetes. The high sugar level is also found in the aqueous humor and this can diffuse into the lens. The sugar is metabolized, and the metabolic products tend to cause the lens to accumulate water electrolytes such as sodium, clouding it. This can be prevented and possibly reversed by vitamin C and naturally occurring yellow pigments called flavonoids, such as quercetin.[157] Flavonoids including quercetin can be found in chocolate, tea, leafy green vegetables, and fruits such as apples, red grapes, and citrus.

By the time a cataract has developed, the lens tissue has deteriorated substantially, so it is not likely to recover with nutritional treatment. Although short-term use of a low level of nutritional supplements is not likely to help much, the available evidence and our knowledge of the causes of cataract suggest that higher doses over a longer period would give a more positive outcome, especially if started in middle age before cataracts are evident.[158] To reduce your chances of developing cataract and many other eye diseases, avoid exposing your eyes for a long time to sunlight, especially when the sun is high in the sky (between 11:00A.M. and 3:00P.M. in the summer). If you're outside in the midday sun for a long time, wear dark glasses that remove UV light and wear a wide-brimmed hat that restricts bright light from the sky. Stop smoking, because it is one of the main risk factors for cataract and many other eye diseases. Eat an excellent diet with lots of dark-green leafy vegetables, and take balanced nutrient supplements that include adequate amounts of antioxidants such as vitamin C (3,000 to 10,000mg per day in divided doses), and vitamin E (400–800IU per day). As you get older, you should increase the nutrient supplements to help protect and maintain your eyes. The risk for cataract is much higher for individuals with diabetes,[159] so it is doubly important to eat an excellent diet with antioxidants such as vitamin C and E and to maintain a low glycemic index in your diet.

Because the lens yellows with age, it is an effective barrier to blue light that would otherwise reach the retina, causing oxidative stress. When the lens is removed in cataract surgery and replaced with a clear plastic lens, paradoxically this increases the amount of blue light and thus the level of oxidative stress on the retina. To prevent this problem, modern plastic lens inserts contain a yellow pigment to remove the blue light.[160]

CHAPTER 5

VITAMINS PREVENT DEGENERATION OF THE PHOTORECEPTORS: RETINAL DETACHMENT, MACULAR DEGENERATION, AND RETINITIS PIGMENTOSA

The rod and cone photoreceptors are essential for vision because they are sensitive to light. But even in a normal eye, they are a weak link. They have one of the highest metabolic rates in the body, and they are delicate and require continuous regeneration, so they are subject to a variety of diseases, most of which are thought to be age-related and caused in part by oxidative stress. Macular degeneration and retinitis pigmentosa are degenerative diseases of photoreceptors, and are linked to other serious health problems such as heart and vascular disease and high blood pressure. The normal retina is only weakly attached to the pigment epithelium and can be detached by physical damage such as a blow to the eye or inflammation. Although detachment can happen in a variety of conditions and diseases of photoreceptors, vitamins and nutrients taken in sufficient amounts can help prevent these diseases.

RETINAL DETACHMENT

In the normal eye, the retina is only weakly attached to the pigment epithelium and can be separated by physical damage such as a blow to the eye or inflammation. In retinas that have diseases such as macular degeneration or diabetic retinopathy, the attachment is weakened so retinal detachment is more common. When this occurs, fluid may accumulate beneath the retina, progressively detaching a larger area from the pigment epithelium. Wherever the retina is detached for more than a few hours from the pigment epithelium, the photoreceptors start to degenerate, and after a few days of detachment, the photoreceptors will start to die.[161] Once such damage has occurred, the remainder of the retinal neurons do not receive normal responses and will eventually degenerate and die as well.[162] For this reason acute retinal detachment is a medical emergency where timely treatment is crucial to preserve sight. If no more than a few days have passed after detachment, an ophthalmologist can save the retina by pulsing a laser to cause small spots of scar tissue in the retina and pigment epithelium that hold the retina in place at the back of the eye.

Although timely laser treatment can reattach the retina, it cannot always reestablish normal vision. After detachment, the retinal pigment epithelium (RPE) cells tend to dedifferentiate, that is, they tend to grow uncontrollably and lose their ability to function as normal RPE cells that contact and care for the photoreceptors.[163] One treatment that seems to help is vitamin C. This helps preserve the RPE cells, preventing their abnormal growth, which helps them contact the photoreceptor outer segments and function normally.[164] A similar treatment that helps preserve RPE cells and prevent retinal detachment is N-acetylcysteine, a precursor for glutathione, a powerful antioxidant.[165] In Eales' disease, retinal blood vessels become inflamed and have abnormal new growth, leading to hemorrhages and sometimes to retinal detachment. In this disease, typically oxidative stress builds up, causing the polyunsaturated fatty acids in photoreceptors and the RPE to become oxidized, and the levels of antioxidants such as vitamin C and E to drop.[166] This suggests that supplements of vitamin C and E could prevent the inflammation, oxidative stress, and likely the progression to retinal detachment. Diabetic retinopathy, which damages retinal blood vessels, sometimes causing their abnormal growth, can cause retinal detachment. This type of retinopathy can be treated by lowering the glycemic index of the diet along with vitamin C and other antioxidants to prevent inflammation and damage (see Diabetic Retinopathy in Chapter 6).

Some common questions ask why the is retina so delicate—why are the photoreceptors so easily pulled away from the RPE and choroid? And why, when the photoreceptors are pulled away from the RPE, do they die within a few days? Although not all the details are known, we do know some important facts. The retina has one of the highest metabolic rates of any organ in the body, and the photoreceptors are responsible for much of this metabolic energy use. In the dark, photoreceptors, especially our 90 million rods, use a tremendous amount of energy because they are continuously generating an electrical current consisting of sodium and calcium ions, called the dark current. When a photon is absorbed, a rod generates a tiny reduction in its dark current. This is then transmitted to second-and third-order neurons and then to the brain. We are thus able to see single photons in the dark. When you are in an unlit room with a window to the outside at night, and you look at a blank wall surface, you can see the single photons as a marked flickering similar to the "snow" on an analog TV set on a blank channel. The photons you see are emitted by street lights, the moon, and stars. They come into the room through the window and reflect back and forth on surfaces around the room until they are absorbed at random by your photoreceptors. This random absorption of just a few photons causes a fluctuation in the perceived light intensity, which is responsible for the flickering you see in the dark. If you look very carefully, you can also see a similar but weaker flickering at all levels of illumination during the day. This originates in biological noise sources in the eye, not from fluctuation in single photon absorption. The photoreceptors are miraculously sensitive, but also very expensive! Bright daylight bleaches all the rhodopsin pigment. The photoreceptors are incapable of repairing themselves, so the pigment must be regenerated every night from vitamin A. They need the RPE cells to digest the worn-out discs that contain bleached rhodopsin, and to secrete fresh rhodopsin that the rods quickly soak up. The RPE cells hold onto the photoreceptors, and for this reason are responsible for holding the retina attached to the back of the eye, where the choroidal matrix of blood vessels are that support the photoreceptors' huge energy requirement. This makes the photoreceptors the high energy luminaries of the eye, but like many movie stars, they require pampering. Oxygen levels in the outer retina and RPE are among the highest in the body, and these levels rise in the day because the photoreceptors utilize less energy with bright light. Because of their high metabolism, they are very susceptible to oxidative damage in their mitochondria, and they are dependent on a complex system of support. If anything goes wrong with this system, the retina can be pulled off the back of the eye when it receives a hard physical shock. When this happens the photoreceptors lose their system of energy and biochemical support from the choroid and RPE. Without this support, they die.

Part of the problem is that the eye is a sphere that rotates very quickly when we move our gaze. Ordinarily, the retina can withstand this rotation, because it is supported on the inside by the vitreous humor, a gel-like viscous liquid. But the retina, being part of a sphere that fits on the inside of the eyeball, is adapted to one particular spherical diameter. If the eye changes diameter quickly, the retina has a big problem. It may get torn or pulled off the back of the eye by physical forces when it can't change shape fast enough. This can happen, for example, when flying in an airplane with sudden changes in pressure, or it may happen when the eye or head is jarred suddenly. If the retina tears, a "bubble" of vitreous can get underneath and push the retina up off the back of the eye, often causing more of the retina to detach. This is more likely to happen in older people or those who have suffered vitreous detachment. It is also more common in patients who have had cataract surgery.

Good nutrition is important in recovering from a detached retina. However, taking adequate amounts of antioxidants throughout our lives is crucial to prevent the buildup of oxidative-stress-induced damage that can cause retinal detachment. If you are in one of the risk categories for retinal detachment such as aging, extreme nearsightedness, eye injury, or a personal or family history of retinal detachment, it is important to have good overall nutrition and an adequate level of nutrients to prevent common deficiencies. Vitamin A is essential, but other common nutrients, such as vitamins B, C, and E; calcium; magnesium; omega-3 oils; zinc; copper; and selenium are also essential for eye health. Because vitamin C is necessary for the synthesis of collagen and also as an antioxidant, it is crucial for eye health. The eye is held together to a large extent by collagen, so it's important to take 1,000-3,000 milligrams (mg) of vitamin C three to five times daily to keep your vitamin C level high.

MACULAR DEGENERATION

Age-related macular degeneration (AMD) is a disease of the retina in which photoreceptors progressively die near the macula, the central region of the eye.[167] AMD is the leading worldwide cause of blindness in people aged fifty years or more.[168] It can be diagnosed fairly easily by direct viewing or photographs of the back of the eye, called viewing the *fundus* (derived from the Latin word for *bottom*). In the "dry" form of AMD, cellular waste deposits are generated between the photoreceptors and the choroid. The waste deposits collect inside RPE cells in granules of *lipofuscin* which comprises the partially digested contents of the photoreceptors' outer segment discs. Underneath the RPE cells near a barrier called "Bruch's membrane;" the waste collects in deposits called *drusen* (derived from the German word for *geode*). Exactly how or why these deposits build up is unknown, but they are thought to be caused by oxidative damage to the retina and pigment epithelium. In the "wet" form of AMD, new blood vessels grow from the choroid at the back of the eye, pushing the retina away from the choroid, tending to cause retinal detachment. Although a large risk factor for AMD is genetic, both forms are thought to be initiated by oxidative damage, consistent with a typical onset after age fifty. Thus, although AMD is considered an incurable age-related disease, it is caused by damage to the eye that can be mitigated by proper nutrition.

AMD is due at least in part to oxidative damage.[169] One of the most important environmental risk factors for AMD is smoking, which causes oxidative damage in many tissues of the eye.[170] In a study of patients with AMD caused by degeneration of photoreceptor outer segments, those who smoked were on average sixty-four years old, whereas those who did not smoke were on average seventy-one years old.[171] Studies of the effects of smoking on AMD have shown a twofold increased risk of AMD, and smoking together with certain genetic mutations increases the risk for AMD up to thirty-fold.[172] Inhaling secondhand smoke is almost as bad as light smoking, because the smoke that emanates from the tip of a cigarette tends to have more toxic chemicals than the exhaled smoke.[173] Some of the toxins present in cigarette smoke are known to induce cell death in the RPE,[174] which is precisely the place in the eye where AMD is thought to initiate.[175] Smoke also induces the expression of VEGF, one of the factors thought responsible for initiating wet AMD.[176] Other important risk factors for AMD are high blood pressure,[177] and exposure to bright sunlight over many years, which is associated with AMD in people with low antixodant levels.[178] Chronic inflammation and problems with the immune system are implicated in the initiation of AMD, and these are also associated with other age-related diseases such as Alzheimer's and atherosclerosis.[179]

One of the typical problems within RPE cells is that lipofuscin, specks of dark yellow pigment from incomplete digestion of fatty cellular debris, along with other oxidized material, form granules inside the RPE cells.[180] The eye is particularly sensitive to age-related disease because the buildup of lipofuscin starts at an early age, even in infancy.[181] The infant's eye is clearer and thus more blue, so more UV light gets transmitted to the retina, causing an early buildup in lipofuscin for those infants who are susceptible. The lipofuscin absorbs light, which generates oxidative stress, causing more lipofuscin buildup. Typically the process then accelerates. Over a person's lifetime the RPE cells get overloaded with lipofuscin granules. The area immediately surrounding the fovea, called the parafoveal ring, where the rod density is highest,[182] is usually the location of the largest accumulation of lipofuscin, and is typically where the degenerative process of the RPE cells starts in AMD.[183] A possible cause for AMD was recently suggested by a study of damage to mitochondrial DNA in RPE cells. Although the DNA of RPE mitochondria is damaged at specific sites by aging, the damage to the RPE genome from AMD is more widespread and more severe.[184] This is consistent with what we know about oxidative stress in the retina. RPE cells must dispose of old discs from the photoreceptor outer segments, which are often highly oxidized. This process can start chemical reaction chains of free radicals within the RPE cells. Their mitochondria contain chromophores that absorb light and generate free radicals, both of which can damage mitochondrial DNA. When damaged cellular debris is concentrated into lipofuscin granules, the chromophores (molecules that absorb light of a certain color) within the granules tend to absorb light, which can cause even more oxidative stress.[185] As early AMD progresses to advanced AMD, the photoreceptors and RPE cells get overwhelmed and eventually the retina becomes dysfunctional or detaches. Once most of the photoreceptors die, the retina "remodels" by disconnecting its synaptic connections, so recovery becomes impossible.[186]

When your ophthalmologist gives you eye drops to dilate your pupil and proceeds to look into your eye with an ophthalmoscope, he or she is looking for anything abnormal, such as cancerous lesions or tears in the retina, but especially any signs of drusen under the retina that may signal progressive retinal degenerative diseases. Drusen are readily visible, and come in two forms: "hard" and "soft."Hard drusen are small, sometimes at the limit of visibility (25 micrometres [μm]), but are fairly common, and are not thought to be directly linked to macular degeneration.[187] Soft drusen are larger with a yellow tint, and may begin to run together to take up most of the area within the macula, which is a sign that macular degeneration is progressing. The fundus view allows a quick check for drusen, but the existence of drusen does not necessarily mean a diagnosis of irreversible progressive macular degeneration.

The good news is that we have accumulated a good deal of knowledge about the stages of AMD and the effects of toxins and light on the risk for AMD, and now grasp its basic causes. We can develop a nutritional program that reduces the risks of developing AMD with this information. We know that antioxidants can help prevent AMD, because a diet containing antioxidants and beneficial nutrients (beta-carotene, vitamins C and E, lutein, zeaxanthin, magnesium, zinc, and copper) is associated with the lowest risk of drusen and advanced AMD.[188]

In the 2001 Age-Related Eye Disease Study, the effect of the supplements was tested in a randomized controlled trial with several thousand participants.[189] Those that received zinc or zinc plus antioxidants had a lower risk for getting both early and advanced AMD, and those that received higher doses of these nutrients had the greatest reduction in risk.[190] Lutein and zeaxanthin have been associated with reduced risk for wet AMD and the buildup of drusen.[191] Although such randomized controlled trials (RCTs) do not tell us the mechanism for the improvement, enough is known about AMD for us to have a fairly good idea of why the treatment works.

We also know that omega-3 fatty acids, available in oily fish, walnuts, and flaxseed oil, are helpful in preventing AMD. A recent study showed that consumption of oily fish and its high content of omega-3 fatty acids DHA and EPA was correlated with a reduced risk of AMD.[192] The reasons behind this are that DHA is essential to the retina and is found in large quantities in the disc membranes of photoreceptor outer segments,[193] where it helps to enhance mobility of the proteins involved in visual transducation (sight), and it is also thought to be involved in regeneration of rhodopsin.[194] People who eat oily fish several times per week have a reduced risk of getting advanced AMD.[195]

Another recent RCT studied the effect of B vitamins, specifically, pyridoxine (vitamin B_6), folate (vitamin B_9), and cobalamin (vitamin B_{12}) on AMD.[196] The study gave different combinations of these vitamins to 5,400 women at risk of heart disease, who were part of an existing RCT for the influence of other vitamins (beta-carotene, vitamin C, and vitamin E) on heart disease. The study gave a combination treatment consisting of folic acid (2.5mg per day), pyridoxine hydrochloride (vitamin B_6) (50mg per day), and cyanocobalamin (vitamin B_{12}) (1mg per day) or a placebo. The study found that taking the B vitamins over a seven-year period reduced the risk of developing AMD by 35 to 40 percent.

The rationale for the beneficial effect of these B vitamins is that AMD is associated with high blood levels of homocysteine, which is an intermediate biochemical in the metabolism of cysteine, an essential amino acid.[197] Homocysteine is elevated after heavy exercise andis thought to be a marker for metabolic stress. It is an important risk factor for blood clots and heart disease.[198] An elevated level of homocysteine damages the inner lining of blood vessels, the endothelium and commonly originates in a deficiency of B vitamins, which is often found in older people.[199] Thus, supplements of these vitamins are likely to maintain and improve the metabolic function of the body's tissues, which will help to reduce the blood level of homocysteine. This helps maintain health of the blood vessels and tissues of the eye and retina, and is a relevant factor in reducing the risk of AMD.[200]

Another way to reduce your risk for AMD is to eat a diet with a low glycemic index (one that moderates the amount of blood sugar and raises it slowly after a meal). Recent studies have found that a high-glycemic-index diet is associated with substantial risk for early AMD.[201] The probable reason for this is that sugar in the bloodstream lessens its antioxidant capacity, and hyperglycemia (high blood sugar) directly causes oxidative stress.[202] For example, some starchy foods, such as refined sugar, rice, and taro, release sugar quickly when digested, and should be avoided. Whole-grain cereals such as rolled oats, taken without much sugar, are known to release sugar slowly. For those who eat a lot of sugar and starch, eating these grains instead tends to lower blood sugar and reduce oxidative stress. And, as described below, it is very important to get the right amount of iron in your diet-not too little and not too much-to lower your risk of macular degeneration and other age-related eye diseases.

The reduction in risk is thought to be greater when the vitamins, antioxidants, and other beneficial nutrients are taken in a sufficient amount along with a varied diet containing vegetables, whole grains, and fruits over many years, preferably over a lifetime.[203] Antioxidants can prevent oxidative-stress-induced damage to arteries in the retina and choroid, which helps to prevent wet AMD. Lutein and zeaxanthin are thought to be directly involved because they form the yellow macular filter, which removes the higher-energy blue wavelengths, lowering the oxidative stress on the macula. In addition, lutein and zeaxanthin are antioxidants that can prevent oxidative stress, and are thought to quench (neutralize) free radicals.[204] A relatively low level of vitamin E (average of 300 international units [IU] per day) produced a small reduction in the risk for AMD, but a greater effect was shown for those who also took multivitamins.[205] The levels of supplements necessary to achieve an optimal reduction in AMD are easy to get, but are not contained in most multivitamin tablets.[206] The level of vitamins C and E in most eye studies has not been high by orthomolecular standards; for example, the vitamin C level of 500mg per day and a vitamin E level of 200–400IU per day typically used in studies is considered low to minimal, and higher levels of these nontoxic antioxidants are very likely beneficial in the long term. Given the low levels of vitamins in the AREDS study, it is remarkable that any benefit was found. But one suspects that levels tenfold higher of these vitamins, which are easily tolerable and nontoxic, would provide even a greater benefit. It seems reasonable to expect that when higher levels are tested in a randomized controlled trial (RCT), the resulting benefits will be even more obvious.

Interestingly but not surprisingly, recent evidence shows that vitamin D is protective against AMD.[207] A study of fundus photographs of 7,700 people across the United States was scored for the presence of drusen and pigment abnormalities, and the level of dietary intake of vitamins and the blood level of vitamin D were noted. The study found that the blood level of vitamin D was inversely related with early AMD. Milk consumption was related to the vitamin D level, presumably because milk is vitamin-D fortified. Additional vitamin D supplements were also helpful in reducing early AMD in the people taking less than one serving of milk per day. Those subjects who did not drink milk or take vitamin D supplements also had an inverse relationship between the blood level of vitamin D and early AMD, implying that vitamin D from exposure to sunlight works to prevent AMD, as long as you get enough. The cause of this robust effect appears to be the ability of vitamin D to prevent inflammation. Vitamin D is known from previous studies to strongly enhance T-suppressor cells, which reduce inflammation caused by the immune system, and it also reduces proinflammatory agents in the body.[208] This is thought to be relevant to preventing the progression of AMD because inflammatory diseases such as gout and emphysema are associated with AMD. Also, a recent study found that AMD is associated with the risk for coronary heart disease.[209] Another study found vitamin D reduces the risk for heart disease, suggesting that the causes of both conditions are similar. Both AMD and heart disease are associated with inflammation, and vitamin D reduces inflammation to produce a beneficial effect.[210]

This research suggests that the increase in risk for developing AMD with age is no coincidence. Light, environmental toxins, and peroxidative agents such as iron cause oxidative damage in the eye, damaging the photoreceptor outer segment discs, and this tends to damage the RPE cells when they recycle the oxidized outer segments. If this oxidative damage to the eye continues, it causes RPE cells to generate internal deposits of lipofuscin, which tend to enlarge when they are exposed to more oxidative stress. The outer segment discs, which are made of fatty acids, contain a large fraction of polyunsaturated fatty acids (omega-3 and omega-6 oils) that are easily oxidized. The discs must be recycled to allow the photoreceptor to regenerate new ones containing a fresh supply of rhodopsin pigment. If the RPE cells are stressed with oxidative damage accumulated from long hours of light exposure, they cannot dispose properly of the oxidized lipids in the lipofuscin granules. The oxidized lipids then continually damage the RPE cells, preventing them from correctly recycling the oxidized material. This process continues and gets worse with age. However, when additional amounts of the omega-3 fatty acids DHA and EPA are given to rats, their outer segment membranes incorporate more of them, resulting in less damage and cell death.[211] A recent study found lower levels of coenzyme Q_{10} (CoQ_{10}) in the eyes of older people who are at risk for age-related eye diseases such as AMD, suggesting that supplementation with this antioxidant can help to prevent age-related eye diseases.

The implications of this nutritional research for preventing AMD are straightforward. You can be proactive by taking nutrients such as the carotenoids lutein and zeaxanthin, the vitamin BS, C, D, and E, omega-3 oils, zinc, and selenium, in sufficient quantity. This can reduce your risk of AMD dramatically. Eat a healthy diet, with plenty of vegetables, and avoid rice, taro, and refined sugar.[212] Each individual has a different glycemic response,[213] so pay attention to the sweet and starchy foods you eat and try to determine which ones raise your blood sugar and make you sleepy after a meal. Wear dark glasses when you are exposed to bright light for many hours to reduce oxidative stress on your eyes, for it is the accumulated damage that appears to be most harmful. Don't take excessive amounts of vitamins, for example vitamin A, because it can cause toxicity at high doses. But do take sufficient amounts of the essential vitamins and nutrients. Because many eye diseases have common origins, the optimal amounts of vitamins and nutrients may be similar for different conditions. But the optimal amounts can also vary widely depending on the individual's needs. We will revisit this issue and discuss the doses in more detail in Chapter 8.

NIGHT BLINDNESS

A variety of problems with the eye can cause difficulty seeing at night. Genetic mutations in the rod pathways can cause them to be dysfunctional. Most of these genetic conditions cannot be treated effectively with current drug technology. A reduction of contrast sensitivity from cataracts can cause low vision at night, because glare from bright lights can obscure low-contrast details. Many night-vision problems can be effectively treated with orthomolecular medicine, however. Night blindness can occur from a lack of vitamin A, which is needed to regenerate the rhodopsin pigment in the rod photoreceptors. This form of night blindness can be prevented by making sure you get enough vitamin A in your diet.

Every time your eyes are exposed to very bright light, for example, from direct sunlight or vehicle headlights, you become temporarily night blind. As described above, the pigment molecule rhodopsin in the outer segments of rod photoreceptors is bleached by light. Therefore the rod pigment is completely bleached when the eyes are exposed to a bright flash of light. The rods must regenerate the pigment in their outer segment discs before you can see in the dark again. If not all the pigment is bleached, some night vision remains. This temporary blindness is normal, and can happen within a few seconds. Depending upon how much pigment is bleached, it may take anywhere from fifteen minutes to an hour for good night vision to return. The discs require vitamin A, omega-3, and omega-6 fatty acids, as well as protein, calcium, and magnesium, and an adequate level of antioxidants for the regeneration process, so any deficiency of these nutrients is likely to contribute to night blindness. An excellent diet can help prevent it.

Oxidative stress and age-related damage to the eye, such as deterioration of the photoreceptors and RPE cells, generates waste products (lipofuscin and drusen) from oxidation of fatty acids. These can cause night blindness symptoms and AMD. For example, too much or too little iron can cause oxidative stress in the eye. In some cases this buildup of oxidized detritus will be cleared by application of polyphenols, such as resveratrol, that remove metal ions.[214] Many genetic diseases can cause rod photoreceptors or other retinal neurons to die or malfunction, causing night blindness. A common type of night blindness is caused by retinitis pigmentosa (see below), in which rods die, causing night blindness at first. Later cones also die, causing a progressive loss of peripheral vision.

Many night-vision problems can be effectively prevented, treated, or reversed with orthomolecular medicine and good nutrition. You can help your body maintain good night vision with an adequate intake of vitamin A or carotene, omega-3 fatty acids found in flaxseed oil and oily fish, and a good overall diet with lots of leafy green vegetables and raw sprouts.

RETINITIS PIGMENTOSA

Another disease of photoreceptors is retinitis pigmentosa (RP), which is a group of night-blindness diseases related to AMD in which rod photoreceptors die, often due to an abnormal mutation in a single gene.[215] In the initial stages, RP causes night blindness and a lack of ability to dark-adapt. The age at which it is first noticed and its progression vary widely. RP is not usually "syndromic"—in other words, it can't be easily recognized by a group of clinical symptoms, because it can be caused by a diversity of different genetic mutations.[216]

Invariably, after the rod photoreceptors die, the cone photoreceptors also progressively die, resulting in gradual blindness, often starting in the periphery of the visual field. Cone death might be caused by a toxin; or the lack of an essential biochemical coming from rods; or by an attack from microglia, which are part of the body's immune defense; or it might be caused directly by oxidative stress or a nutritional deficiency.[217]

Stargardt's disease is similar to RP in that it is a photoreceptor degeneration caused by an abnormal mutation in a gene, usually in the first two decades of life, that indirectly causes buildup of oxidized lipofuscin detritus.[218] Oxidative stress in retinitis pigmentosa is thought to originate, as in macular degeneration, from free radicals generated by light, possibly through an effect on vasculature. Therefore, limiting exposure to light is thought to slow progression of the damage to photoreceptors.[219] The damage is thought to spread through oxidative damage to lipids.[220]

Once most of the photoreceptors die, the retina has little chance to provide vision, even though some cones survive. The reason is that the second layer of neurons, the bipolar and horizontal cells, depend on visual input for their synaptic connections. Without rods and cones to provide a chemical signal, the dendritic branches of the bipolar and horizontal cells start to migrate as if in search of the visual input that they are supposed to process. The dendrites of the bipolar and horizontal cells regrow and make aberrant synaptic connections. Often the blood vessels start growing again, leading to other problems. The result is that the neurons of the retina "remodel" their circuitry so that it no longer functions normally.[221] Thus, while the retina can survive photoreceptor death, it is no longer viable for sight.

If cone death could be prevented, patients with retinitis pigmentosa could still read and live independently. For this reason many studies have focused on slowing cone death. Although the night blindness symptoms can start early in life, the progression to cone death and complete blindness is often gradual, over a period of decades. It is not currently known why the cones may survive in some cases for years after the rods die. If the mutations that initiate RP were acutely lethal one would imagine the cones would die quickly early in life, soon after the rods. For example, if the cones die because of a toxin emitted from the dying rods, one would hypothesize that cones should die immediately after the rods.[222] However, after the rods die off, the cones sometimes survive for years, which tends to discount the toxin hypothesis.

The slow progression of RP appears to be due to biochemical problems that build up with age, which suggests that a variety of RP types caused by different genetic makeup can be addressed with nutritional supplements.[223] Compared to rods, the cones are scarcer and therefore use less oxygen. Many blood vessels throughout the body and in the eye are "autoregulated;"that is, they regulate the blood flow to maintain a relatively constant level of oxygen for the tissues surrounding them.[224] Choroidal blood vessels do not autoregulate in this way, however, so after the rods die in RP, the cones continue to receive the same high level of oxygenation from the choroidal blood vessels and thus are subject to increased oxidative stress.[225] One hypothesis states that a critical period exists, in which the photoreceptors that die early in RP do so because of an inability to utilize oxygen. Then, later in the disease, the photoreceptors become hypersensitive to oxygen and die from oxidative stress.[226] This suggests that if rod death could be slowed, the surviving rods and cones would have less oxidative stress. One focus of research in RP has been to prevent oxidative stress with nutrition to explore this theory.

A recent study of an RP-like genetic disease in mice showed that once the rods die, the cones lose a protective biochemical that ordinarily acts as an antioxidant to protect them from the high levels of oxygen found in the retina.[227] In another study, a higher level of insulin allowed the cones to survive longer, and a lower level quickened their demise, leading to the hypothesis that cones finally succumb to a nutritional deficiency, as if they essentially starve to death.[228] The study suggested that with such a nutritional deficiency, the outer segments cannot grow as fast, and they can't absorb as much glucose and other nutrients, further aggravating the problem. Thus suggests that nutritional supplements will help to prevent cone death.

However, the evidence from some RCTs on treating RP with nutritional supplements has not always been clear.[229] The studies focused on specific combinations and doses, and their conclusions are specific to those doses. When the conclusions differ from what was expected, they are difficult to generalize. In studies testing the effect of a single supplementary nutrient on the progression of cone death in RP, the results have not always shown definite improvements depending on what doses and combinations of supplements are given, and thus it is difficult to know what specific combinations of supplements are helpful. The results for one study of treatment of RP with vitamin A and 400IU per day of vitamin E appeared to show that the vitamin E treatment accelerated the loss of photoreceptors.[230] One possible cause for this effect is the tendency for vitamin E to strengthen blood vessels, slow clotting, and promote blood flow.[231] This suggested, paradoxically, that what is good for the health of arteries and for circulation of the blood may increase oxidative stress for a retina that has been damaged by the loss of most of its photoreceptors. Another possible cause of this effect is that vitamin E tends to slow the growth of RPE cells, which is helpful in some retinal diseases such as diabetic retinopathy but not for RP, where growth of the RPE cells is helpful for the photoreceptors.[232] However, another perspective on this issue is that some types of RP can apparently be caused by a lack of vitamin E. People with a type of genetic abnormality that prevents vitamin E uptake are prone to RP.[233] The patients had several neurological problems, and had a buildup of lipofucsin in the eye, supporting the oxidative stress hypothesis. In this case, a vitamin E supplement (400–900IU per day) was reported to prevent progression of the RP symptoms.[234]

Damage from oxidative stress occurs typically throughout cells, in their membranes, cytoplasm, and in subcellular organelles. In some studies, short-term supplementation with a water-soluble (hydrophilic) or fat-soluble (lipophilic) antioxidant alone seems relatively ineffective in treating RP, because oxidative damage can be found in both lipophilic and hydrophilic compartments. This suggests that to be most helpful in preventing RP, a combination of a variety of dietary antioxidants, both water-soluble like vitamin C, and fat-soluble like vitamin E, should be given over a period of several decades. This will allow the natural transporters in the blood-retina barrier to counteract the long-term damage that genetic mutations tend to generate.

There is abundant evidence that an excellent diet, along with a combination of antioxidants and other essential nutrients widely understood to benefit overall health, will slow the deterioration of photoreceptors in some types of RP.[235] Essential nutrients such as vitamin A, vitamin C, vitamin E, and omega-3 fatty acids can slow or prevent the damage to photoreceptors and their RPE and choroidal support system in some types of RP.[236] In case studies, a supplement of thiamine (vitamin B_1) reversed an acute anemia with RP.[237] In a mouse model of RP, a supplement of vitamins C and E, alpha-lipoic acid, and other antioxidants reduced cone-cell death and slowed rod death.[238] Supplementation with lutein and zeaxanthin, which absorb blue light and have an antioxidant function, slowed the progression of RP.[239] Painkiller drugs that affect mitochondrial function are thought to cause oxidative stress that may contribute to RP and other ocular diseases.[240] Depending on which genes are affected, vitamin A supplements (15,000IU per day) can delay loss of cone function in RP to preserve sight.[241] When lutein (12mg per day) was given in addition, it further reduced the rate of vision loss.[242] A likely cause of this benefit is the necessary role of vitamin A in regenerating the optic pigment. The addition of omega-3 fatty acids such as DHA (1,200mg per day) along with vitamin A (15,000IU per day) was also beneficial.[243] Although these studies were relatively short, typically four to six years, the benefit of these essential nutrient supplements is likely to accumulate over decades, especially if started as a young adult.[244]

Prevention and Treatment of Retinitis Pigmentosa

Overall, it appears that there is very good reason for hope in the early stages of retinitis pigmentosa. If the signs of RP are detected early, before cone function has deteriorated much, nutrition treatments can help to prevent further deterioration. As in the example in Chapter 1, the best nutritional treatment starts with an excellent diet consisting of lots of raw vegetables such as sprouts, dark green leafy vegetables, orange and yellow vegetables such as carrots and sweet potatoes, a modest amount of chicken or red meat, lots of fresh fruits, and other healthy foods such as yogurt. To make sure you are getting enough of the nutrients that have been shown to benefit photoreceptor health, supplement with vitamin A (10,000IU per day), lutein and zeaxanthin (20mg per day), vitamin C (5,000–15,000mg per day in divided doses), and omega-3 fatty acids (ALA/LNA, EPA, DHA 2,000–5,000mg per day). While you're doing this you'll probably want to supplement with other essential nutrients such as vitamin D (3,000–10,000IU per day), calcium (500–1,000mg per day), magnesium (300–600mg per day), and zinc (20–50mg per day) for optimal eye (and body) health. If you suspect that you have a genetic abnormality that puts you at risk for RP, but don't have night blindness or other explicit RP symptoms, you should also consider supplementing with vitamin

E (400–800IU per day, mixed tocopherals and tocotrienols) for best photoreceptor health. For smokers, this nutrition can help to prevent RP, but only if you stop smoking.[245] The assault from the chemicals in smoke damages eye tissues, especially the retina, from oxidative stress. Also, wear dark glasses when you're outside for more than a few minutes. This lifestyle, along with regular consultations with your eye doctor, should help keep you in the best health.

The late stages of retinitis pigmentosa are difficult to treat, because by then the retina has already started to become dysfunctional beyond repair. It appears that the best advice for retaining cone function in late RP is to eat an excellent diet, with supplements of the essential nutrients as mentioned above, but to avoid high doses of vitamin E. Take a multivitamin tablet that contains vitamin E (50–100IU per day), but no additional vitamin E tablet. As always, if you have any special problems such as other eye conditions, high blood pressure, reduced kidney function, or any unusual health problems, you should discuss your diet with a medical professional.

CHAPTER 6

VITAMINS PREVENT DEGENERATION OF RETINAL GANGLION CELLS: GLAUCOMA, DIABETIC RETINOPATHY

Another set of eye diseases of the retinal neurons is caused by damage to the ganglion cells. These nerve cells receive visual signals relayed from the photoreceptors and generate action potentials (spikes) that code our vision into digital impulses, which they send along their axons to the brain. The axons traverse the inner surface of the retina and exit the eyeball at the optic disk. There they join to form the optic nerve and travel several inches to the brainstem. Ganglion cells are subject to oxidative stress similar to photoreceptors, but because their axons project through the optic disk, they have another set of weaknesses, which can cause the diseases described in this chapter.

GLAUCOMA

Glaucoma is a progressive disease of the eye in which the nerve cells that send visual signals to the brain degenerate and gradually die. It is often too late to preserve sight by the time this problem is noticed. Glaucoma is a leading cause of blindness worldwide. It is usually associated with high pressure inside the eyeball, which pinches the axons of the ganglion cells where they exit the eyeball. The pressure in the eye is created by fluid pumped into the eye from the bloodstream. The fluid pressure is drained by small canals around the edge of the iris (Figure 6.1). When the trabecular meshwork, the tissue that covers the canals, gets blocked, the intraocular pressure increases and the optic nerve gets damaged. Open-angle glaucoma, the most common type, is primarily caused by blockage of the trabecular meshwork.

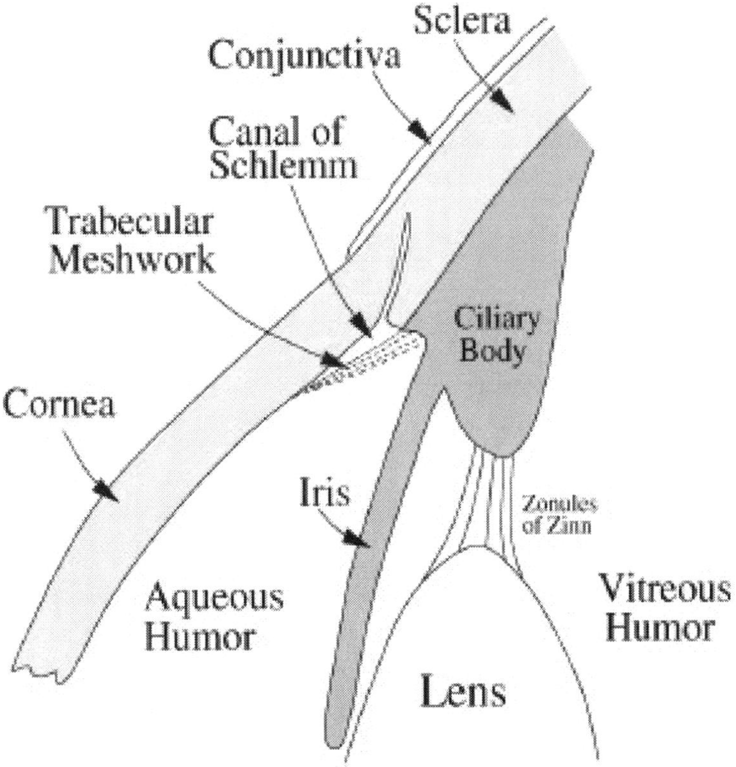

Figure 6.1. Tissues involved in initiating glaucoma, in a horizontal section through the angle of the eye (confluence of the cornea, sclera, ciliary body, and iris), showing the trabecular meshwork and canal of Schlemm. The vitreous humor is under pressure that originates in the bloodstream. Pressure inside the eyeball (sclera and cornea) is necessary to maintain its shape. Normally, the pressure flows from the vitreous humor around the lens into the aqueous humor. To regulate the pressure, the aqueous humor drains into a circular canal around the edge of the iris, called the Ca al of Schlemm, and from there into a series of small veins. The drainage passes through the trabecular meshwork, which can get blocked by debris from the aqueous and vitreous humors that are sloughed off from the tissues inside the eye. In open-angle glaucoma, the trabecular meshwork may be damaged by oxidative stress when the debris that it removes from the drainage contains free radicals, thus limiting its ability to clear the debris. When the trabecular meshwork gets clogged the

intraocular pressure builds up. This causes blockage of the retinal artery where it exits the eye at the optic disk and damages the optic nerve and retina. In closed angle glaucoma, the iris contacts the lens and the trabecular meshwork, which prevents the flow of pressure from the vitreous into the aqueous humor and its drainage through the trabecular meshwork. In dry-eye glaucoma, the conjunctiva (the transparent tissue covering the sclera and the inside of the eyelid) becomes dry and inflamed.

In closed-angle glaucoma, the trabecular meshwork and canals can also be blocked by the iris, which may press against the lens, preventing drainage from the vitreous humor into the aqueous humor. Closed-angle glaucoma often develops quickly and can be acutely painful, so patients usually seek immediate medical attention. However, open-angle glaucoma typically progresses for many years without pain or other symptoms. Normal-tension glaucoma causes a similar type of damage to the optic nerve but is not associated with high pressure in the eyeball. It is thought to be caused by unusually fragile axons, or restricted blood flow, in the optic nerve. A relatively rare type of glaucoma, neovascular glaucoma, occurs when new blood vessels grow near the trabecular meshwork, blocking the drainage into the canal of Schlemm. It is common among those with diabetic retinopathy or those with poor blood flow.

Studies on the factors that initiate glaucoma are focused on two locations in the eye: the arteries that enter the back of the eye through the optic nerve, and the drainage canals at the edge of the iris that are important for regulating intraocular pressure. Because most types of glaucoma are thought to start with high intraocular pressure, any action that reduces pressure would give an immediate benefit. Damage to the retinal arteries is thought to reduce their ability to regulate blood flow, which tends to worsen the pressure buildup inside the eye. This problem is especially serious with atherosclerosis and age-related diseases that cause high blood pressure and associated damage to the arterial walls. When the eye's arteries are unable to regulate their blood pressure, intraocular pressure tends to increase, which reduces their blood flow and therefore their ability to deliver nutrients. This in turn further reduces the ability of the arteries to regulate flow, and further compounds the damage.[246] Thus, to prevent further damage, it is important to maintain blood flow and control intraocular pressure. Vitamin C (3,000 to 10,000 milligrams [mg] per day) and vitamin E (400 to 800 international units [IU] per day) are known to preserve blood vessel function when taken together, and so are likely to help prevent damage typically found in glaucoma.

In all types of glaucoma, damage to the axons of retinal ganglion cells causes them to progressively degenerate. Oxidative stress is thought to be a common component in the degeneration of ganglion cells in glaucoma.[247] Patients with neovascular glaucoma have severe oxidative stress with low levels of vitamin C in the aqueous humor,[248] and the same is true of normal-tension glaucoma, suggesting that a low level of vitamin C inside the eye contributes to glaucoma.[249] Oxidative stress has been shown in the axons of animal models of glaucoma, and free-radical scavengers can prevent retinal ganglion cell death.[250] The damage to the axons may be worsened with high intraocular pressure.[251] The high pressure pinches the central artery of the optic nerve supplying the retinal neurons. This can disrupt the microcirculation of blood flow within the optic nerve and retina. When blood flow is disrupted in this way, the neurons in the retina cannot maintain themselves. Their internal metabolism and the maintenance of the proteins that support the cell's function are halted.[252] The ganglion cells are thought to die at different times during the progression of glaucoma because they receive differing secondary insults, including oxidative stress from light.[253]

The drainage canals that normally regulate intraocular pressure can be blocked by debris from degenerating eye tissue, especially the retina, iris, and lens, due to oxidative damage from light absorption (Figure 6.1). The debris is carried to the trabecular meshwork covering the canals, where it can clog and allow the pressure to build. In a randomized study looking for signs of a high level of debris in the aqueous humor, called "exfoliation syndrome;" those who ate lots of fiber-rich yellow and green vegetables had less exfoliation of debris and also lower intraocular pressure, suggesting that antioxidants can reduce the risk for glaucoma.[254] The trabecular meshwork is also directly affected by oxidative stress, which damages the meshwork cells and their DNA and leads to further oxidative stress and damage.[255] This oxidative stress can be countered very effectively with antioxidants such as vitamins C and E, lutein, and glutathione. In open-angle glaucoma, the mitochondria, which are responsible for energy production inside cells, are thought to be damaged by oxidative stress in cells of the trabecular meshwork.

The standard treatment for glaucoma is to lower the intraocular pressure, and although medical professionals often advise the use of drugs or laser surgery for this purpose, any method that gets the pressure down, including nutrition, is likely to help. Magnesium, found in green vegetables, whole grains, and beans, helps to reduce blood pressure.[256] Chocolate contains a generous amount of magnesium and other substances helpful in lowering intraocular pressure.[257] In normal-tension glaucoma, supplemental magnesium may allow the blood vessels supplying the optic nerve to relax, increasing its blood supply.

A high level of vitamin C (for example, 3,000 to 10,000mg per day or higher, to bowel tolerance) is very effective at reducing intraocular pressure.[258] One reason for the pressure reduction is thought to be its osmotic effect.[259] However, other mechanisms are likely, such as reduction of inflammation and slowing the oxidation of lipids in cell membranes. This prevents cell debris in the vitreous and aqueous humor, which increases outflow through the trabecular mesh and canals that drain the eye.[260]

It is currently hypothesized that increasing the supply of energy can increase ganglion cell survival. One way to achieve this is with antioxidants that scavenge free radicals generated by light and oxidative stress.[261] Another way appears to be to eat a variety of nutrients in an excellent diet. In an observational study of older women lasting ten years, the risk for glaucoma was reduced by 50 percent to 70 percent for those who ate green collards, kale, carrots, or peaches.[262] Underscoring the importance of excellent nutrition, even one serving a month of collards or kale greatly reduced the risk for glaucoma. Although these vegetables contain some vitamin C, a benefit of vitamin C for reducing risk of glaucoma was not observed in this study. The reason is likely that the amount of vitamin C these vegetables contain in a small serving is insufficient for the body's needs.[263] But the authors noted that many other helpful nutrients in these vegetables, such as vitamin A, beta-carotene, vitamin B_2, flavonoids, isothiocyanates, fiber, and potassium were associated with reduced glaucoma risk. They pointed out that antioxidants are likely to be synergistic along with other nutrients present in fruits and vegetables.[264] The precise mechanism by which these nutrients can reduce the risk is not known, but overall it is clear that good nutrition is essential in preventing glaucoma and many other eye diseases.

Levels of ascorbate and other antioxidants such as glutathione are lower inside the eye in glaucoma, suggesting that they are protective against damage.[265] To further preserve ganglion cells under oxidative stress, oral supplements such as lipoic acid, niacinamide (vitamin B_3), and creatinine, are thought to be helpful for enhancing mitochondrial function.[266] Although glaucoma is not considered to be a vitamin-deficiency disease, vitamin E is known be an important regulator of the oxidative damage that causes glaucoma.[267] Vitamin E can delay the onset of glaucoma symptoms in retinal blood vessels,[268] and in a rat model of glaucoma, a vitamin-E deficiency aggravates ganglion cell death, presumably due to a lack of free-radical scavenging.[269]

DIABETIC RETINOPATHY

Diabetes is caused by an inability to utilize blood sugar (glucose), which damages tissues throughout the body. Normally the pancreas secretes insulin into the bloodstream, which causes cells of most tissues to take up glucose. However, in diabetes the tissues don't take up blood sugar normally and the level of blood sugar increases to an excessive level, causing a condition called hyperglycemia. Individuals who are overweight are at a higher risk of diabetes. Type 1 diabetes, which is relatively uncommon, can occur from a genetic problem that causes an inability to make insulin, although the tissues can respond appropriately by taking up sugar once insulin is given. Type 2 diabetes is caused by insulin resistance, in which the body tissues do not take up blood sugar at the normal rate when insulin is released. Both types of diabetes are often treated with insulin injections. The rise of blood sugar in diabetes is thought to be responsible for damaging blood vessels, and it causes oxidative stress.[270] This is a continual problem for the retina because it is exposed to further oxidative stress daily from bright light and environmental toxins.

Diabetic retinopathy can result from the high blood sugar of diabetes in several ways. The retina does not respond to insulin, so it is especially susceptible to diabetes and the oxidative damage caused by high blood sugar. Typically, the retinal damage is greater the longer the patient has diabetes.[271] Hyperglycemia can directly cause damage by a chemical reaction between sugar and either a protein or a lipid molecule. The high level of sugar can cause the metabolic pathways of cells to malfunction because of oxidative stress.[272] The damage from diabetes can cause impaired regulation of iron in the retina. Oxidative stress from diabetes can damage the arteries, which dramatically increases the risk of hemorrhagic stroke.[273] Hemorrhages in the capillaries can release hemoglobin into the retina, and hemoglobin can be damaged by high blood sugar, leading to release of iron. Because iron is a pro-oxidant, this can further increase damage from oxidative stress.[274] All of these pathways caused by the complications of diabetes lead to oxidative stress in the eye and prevent the biochemical machinery in neurons from functioning normally. Retinal damage is, therefore, one of the most common complications of diabetes.[275]

Many studies have shown that antioxidants, including vitamin C, vitamin D, vitamin E, and alpha-lipoic acid, and mineral nutrients such as magnesium and zinc can reduce or prevent retinal damage from diabetes. A higher vitamin C level in the blood reduces the risk for diabetes, likely by reducing oxidative stress.[276] A diet high in fat, often associated with being overweight, reduces the level of vitamin C in the brain, which will tend to increase the risk of damage to the retina.[277] Long-term treatment with antioxidants such as vitamins C, E, and selenium was shown to increase the elasticity of arteries and to reduce blood pressure.[278] Because damage to capillaries is directly linked to diabetic retinopathy, this implies that these antioxidants will help when taken over at least several months to years.

Vitamins and antioxidants have a variety of beneficial effects for diabetic patients. Alpha-lipoic acid (600mg per day) can increase insulin sensitivity in type 2 diabetes, as can chromium supplements (200 to 1,000 micrograms [mcg] per day).[279] Vitamin C (800 to 3,000mg per day), and vitamin E (200 to 1,000IU per day) can help to prevent oxidative stress in diabetes. They can improve blood flow, and lower blood sugar, blood pressure, and cholesterol, all useful in preventing or reversing diabetic retinopathy.[280] Because vitamin C is necessary for synthesis of collagen, an adequate level of vitamin C can reduce the bleeding from retinal capillaries that is typical in diabetes.[281] In a recent randomized controlled trial (RCT), high doses of vitamin D (single one-time doses of 100,000 or 200,000IU) This significantly lowered the systolic (peak) blood pressure of people with type 2 diabetes.[282] is important to prevent retinopathy, because high blood pressure is known to damage retinal blood vessels. Of course, for most adults such huge single doses of vitamin D are unnecessary, because the normal daily dose of 3,000–10,000IU (depending on body mass index and weight) is equivalent and preferable. In addition, several observational studies showed that type 2 diabetes patients with the most severe retinopathy over several decades had the lowest levels of magnesium.[283] While this type of evidence shows a correlation, it does not prove that low magnesium is a cause for the damage. However, magnesium is known to be involved in allowing arteries to relax, lowering blood pressure and improving many other aspects of health.[284] Overall, this suggests that magnesium supplements can lower the risk for retinopathy.

Many studies have shown that exercise and an excellent diet with lots of fruits and vegetables can lower blood sugar and greatly reduce the risk of type 2 diabetes and its associated complications,[285] implying this is effective for preventing diabetic retinopathy. To find out more about this method of treating diabetes and its complications, many popular books are available that explain what can be done to prevent and reverse diabetes, with dietary and exercise methods.[286] With knowledge about how essential vitamins and nutrients can help to prevent diabetes and its risk for diabetic retinopathy, there is considerable hope for diet and nutritional supplements to minimize eye damage.

CHAPTER 7

VITAMINS FOR OTHER CONDITIONS AND DISEASES OF THE EYE

This chapter describes a variety of common eye problems. Most of these are not age-related or serious enough to cause blindness, and can be treated or ameliorated effectively with proper nutrition.

DRY EYE, CONJUNCTIVITIS

Tears, released from the lacrimal glands in the eyelid, are important for lubricating the eye and preventing inflammation and infection. Dry-eye syndrome results when the quantity of tears is insufficient to keep the eye lubricated. This syndrome causes irritation of the cornea, the tissue at the front of the eye, and the conjunctiva, the transparent tissue covering the white scleral tissue at the sides and back of the eyeball. It is sometimes associated with sicca syndrome, an autoimmune disease, but it often occurs in people who are otherwise healthy. Dry eye can be caused by a lack of vitamin A, which is necessary for health of the epithelial cells. These cells generate the mucus that mixes with tears to lubricate the eye.[287]

In one study, topical application of vitamin A drops improved dry eye significantly, even when compared to a widely used drug.[288] Vitamin A has helped people with dry eye from a variety of causes, such as keratoconjunctivis (inflammation of the cornea and conjunctiva), xerophthalmia (a deficiency of tears), or contact-lens-induced dry eye.[289] In some cases, inflammation in the lacrimal glands and the conjunctiva is chronic, and anti-inflammatory treatments are thought to help. Omega-3 (linolenic) and omega-6 (linoleic) fatty acids, taken along with vitamins C and B_6 1 may help because they are pre-cursors of prostaglandin E1[290]. A deficiency of vitamin B_6 caused dry eye in guinea pigs, suggesting that for people with a marginal vitamin B_6 deficiency, a supplement (10–50 milligrams [mg] per day) might help. Similarly, a multivitamin-mineral tablet, containing vitamins C, E, and B_6; zinc; and selenium helped to improve dry eye and boost the immune system,[291] and eye drops containing antioxidants are widely used and are effective.[292]

Conjunctivitis is an inflammation of the conjunctiva on the outside of the eyeball and can include redness and irritation. It has been effectively treated with topical vitamin C (sterile, buffered), and also with oral vitamin C and vitamin A. In other cases, vitamin B_2 and B_3, and B_5 have helped alleviate symptoms and heal the epithelial tissues. In cases where contact lenses have caused conjunctivitis, topical vitamin A drops have been effective.[293]

UVEITIS

Uveitis is an inflammation of the interior of the eye. If it is severe it can lead to blindness. Uveitis can be caused by a variety of problems, such as allergy, infection, or autoimmune disease. Antioxidants are thought to help prevent inflammation in the eye, and a variety of antioxidants are currently being tested in the treatment of uveitis.[294] A recent laboratory study showed that retinoic acid, a metabolic product of vitamin A, helped to prevent autoimmune uveitis.[295] Vitamin C is known to attenuate the symptoms of allergies,[296] and vitamin C and E are thought to help alleviate uveitis because they are antiinflammatory.[297] Eye drops containing buffered vitamin C and/or vitamin E may be helpful to deliver these essential antioxidants to the inflamed region.

CORNEAL ULCERS, CORNEAL TRANSPLANT

The cornea is composed mostly of collagen that remains transparent throughout life. It can be damaged easily, by objects flying into the eye or by a variety of conditions that prevent its cells from maintaining themselves. When it is damaged the cornea is prone to "melting," a condition in which it becomes mushy and weakens due to loss of cross-linking between its collagen fibers.[298] This can cause ulcers in the cornea. This typically occurs in several diseases, for example, in keratoconus, in which the cornea's shape is altered, causing vision to blur. One recent treatment for this condition is to apply eye drops that contain riboflavin (vitamin B_2), after which the cornea is irradiated with ultraviolet (UVA) light, causing the riboflavin to form new cross-links between the collagen fibers. This treatment can temporarily damage the corneal tissue,[299] and it typically requires removal of the corneal epithelium, the surface layer of cells, a process that may allow infections to take hold. In corneal transplants, new corneal tissue is applied to a damaged cornea, but healing is difficult because the cornea is not directly supported by blood vessels. However, vitamins can help.

Vitamin C and amino acids, taken orally, improved the recovery from surgery for corneal ulcers.[300] Vitamin C also helps to prevent corneal ulcers after acid and alkali burns of the cornea.[301] The reason is that vitamin C is required for the synthesis and maintenance of collagen, and it tends to prevent inflammation. Vitamin C helps corneal fibroblast cells synthesize and build up the extracellular matrix of of collagen.[302] In another study, vitamin A, vitamin C, and vitamin E helped mouse corneal tissue survive oxidative stress, suggesting that supplementation with these vitamins can help the cornea recover from injury.[303] Another cause of corneal ulcers is a deficiency of vitamin A. Although this is rare, it can be serious, for example, in cases of anorexia nervosa where the dietary intake of nutrients, including vitamin A, is restricted.[304] A diet with vegetables containing vitamin A and/or supplements can prevent or reverse the corneal damage if it is started before the ulcers are severe.

EYE HERPES, ZOSTER, AND SHINGLES

Several types of virus can attack the eye. They are often treated with steroids or antiviral drugs. Herpes viruses can cause uveitis, conjunctivitis, as well as "red eye." Herpes zoster (chickenpox) can cause shingles in the eye, which can be painful and can lead to more serious eye problems.[305] Viruses can be treated with vitamin C using eye drops containing buffered ascorbate, or taken orally (3,000–50,000mg per day in divided doses, to bowel tolerance), or via an intravenous [IV] line (3,000mg per day).[306] Treatment should continue as long as symptoms remain, and then for an additional twenty-four hours. Vitamin D is known to strengthen the immune system and can help prevent viral infections (5,000–10,000 international units [IU] per day).[307] If you suspect you are low in vitamin D, you should get a blood test. To raise your level of vitamin D quickly, you can take a higher dose (20,000–50,000IU per day) for a few days, under the care of a medical professional. This may help to combat an acute infection.

EYE TWITCH

A variety of conditions can cause eye twitching. The muscles of the eye and eyelid are controlled by nerves from the midbrain, and they are susceptible to vitamin and nutrient deficiencies, and also to fatigue, stress, eye strain, irritation of the cornea, or lack of sleep. A deficiency of calcium and/or magnesium is known to produce eye twitching, as is a borderline deficiency of vitamin B_{12}[308] A common treatment for this problem is to try a multivitamin tablet along with additional supplements of calcium and magnesium supplement (chelate, malate, or chloride), which may solve the problem in a few weeks. Another treatment that has helped some patients is lecithin, which contains choline, a precursor for the neurotransmitter acetyl-choline. It also contains phospholipids that are used to maintain membranes of neurons in the brain. Last, because eye twitch is often related to stress and stimulation, it may help to work actively to reduce your level of stress and to reduce your intake of caffeine and other stimulants. If your twitches persist, you should see a doctor.

VITREOUS FLOATERS, VITREOUS DETACHMENT, MACULAR HOLE, RETINAL TEARING

Floaters are small objects that are suspended in the liquid gel of the vitreous humor in front of the retina. The vitreous is a gelatinous liquid, consisting mostly of water, that contains fibers connecting it to the back of the eye. The floaters are perceived as gray silhouettelike objects that cast an out-of-focus shadow and move to some extent when the eye moves. When the tissues inside the eye become weak, typically after fifty years of age, some of the fibers and cells break off from the inside of the eyeball and float around in the vitreous. The vitreous fibers are composed of collagen and hyaluronic acid, and are connected to the inner limiting membrane of the retina.[309] They are susceptible to damage, especially when the eyeball is rotated quickly, as when following a fast-moving object with the eyes.[310] Vitreous detachment means that the vitreous fibers have broken, often contracting to pull away from the retina, with the space between filling with liquid. This can occur early in life over a small portion of the retina, and may progress very slowly with age, without any obvious symptoms, until complete detachment occurs.[311] Individuals with myopia are more likely to have early vitreous detachment.[312]

In older individuals, the vitreous gel and its fibers tend to shrink, the vitreous gets more viscous and stringy, and the space between the shrunken vitreous gel and the retina, which is filled with vitreous fluid, enlarges. When the vitreous shrinks, the fibers can break and cause vitreous detachment or they can pull on the retina and cause a retinal tear. When a tear happens, the vitreous fluid can go inside the inner limiting membrane and cause a small retinal detachment.[313] When this happens, it is often in the macula, and is sometimes called a macular hole.

Although floaters can be evident at any time, early or late in life, they do not necessarily indicate any damage to the vitreous fibers or the retina. However, a sudden onset of floaters can indicate a vitreous detachment, retinal detachment, or vitreous hemorrhage, and should be checked by an ophthalmologist. Floaters can be alarming to those unfamiliar with them, but they usually disappear within a few weeks or months.

Although ophthalmologists typically focus on managing acute problems and try to anticipate and react quickly to events that could indicate retinal detachment, preventive treatment may be more effective if it is initiated early in life. Because the vitreous fibers contain several forms of collagen, a potential treatment is vitamin C, which is concentrated in the vitreous, preventing oxidation and helping to maintain the vitreous fiber collagen. A typical dose is 3,000–10,000mg per day, to bowel tolerance. For long-term prevention, vitamin C can be taken along with vitamin A/beta-carotene, vitamin E, alpha-lipoic acid, zinc, and selenium. Hyaluronic acid is part of the extracellular matrix, and is found in many places in the body including the skin and synovial fluid of joints. It is also involved in initiating and moderating inflammation and wound repair.[314] A precursor to hyaluronic acid in the vitreous is Nacetyl-glucosamine. This suggests that supplements of N-acetyl-glucosamine may help keep the vitreous from degradation.

OPTIC NEURITIS

Optic neuritis is an inflammation of the optic nerve that carries visual information from the eye to the brain. It comprises the axons of ganglion cells, which course over the surface of the retina and exit the eyeball at the optic disk (blind spot), sending visual information to the brain. Partial or total blindness can result when inflammation of the optic nerve is severe. A common cause for optic neuritis is multiple sclerosis (MS), which is an inflammation of the myelin sheath that covers the axons of nerve cells in the brain, spinal cord, and the eye.[315] Although optic neuritis from MS is almost always painful, the optic neuritis symptoms of MS do not necessarily reflect a worsening of long-term MS symptoms.[316] Other causes for optic neuritis are stroke, syphilis, encephalitis, meningitis, and neuromyelitis optica, which is thought to be a related type of autoimmune disease.[317] Recently it was shown that the incidence of MS episodes was inversely proportional to the amount of vitamin D in the blood.[318] This implies that MS and its manifestation as optic neuritis can be treated with adequate vitamin D (5,000–10,000IU per day). A standard blood test for vitamin D (25-hydroxyvitamin D, abbreviated 25-OH-D) is available at any blood laboratory, and for optimal health it is best to raise the blood level to at least 50 nanograms (ng) per milliliter (ml). In addition, viral infections such as viral encephalitis can be treated with high doses of vitamin C (10,000 to 50,000mg per day).[319] Ischemic stroke, in which a blood clot blocks arteries such as those serving the optic nerve, can be prevented and reversed to some extent by vitamins C and E, and vitamins C, D, and E can help to strengthen the immune system and prevent autoimmune diseases (see Chapter 8).

OCULAR STROKES

A stroke can be caused by blockage of an artery or capillary, for example by a blood clot (ischemic stroke), or by blood leakage (hemorrhagic stroke). Strokes can happen in the eye, for example, a clot can block a retinal artery. When this happens a small part of the retina becomes dysfunctional, and vision is lost within that region. If you look at a large plain object, such as a wall painted with a light color, and you see a dark area that moves with your gaze, you may have had an ocular stroke. In some cases a healing process allows normal vision to reappear in the affected area after several months.

An ischemic stroke can be prevented and in some cases reversed by vitamin C and vitamin E, and a hemorrhagic stroke can be prevented with vitamin C and vitamin E taken long term.[320] These vitamins strengthen the arteries. Vitamin C helps to maintain the strength of collagen in the arteries and to keep them elastic,[321] and vitamin E helps to prevent inflammation in arteries and dissolves clots.[322] Thus, when taken together, vitamin C and vitamin E tend to strengthen blood vessels and prevent strokes.

RECOVERY FROM EYE SURGERY

Surgery causes an acute reaction, similar to an injury, that includes an immune response, inflammation, recruitment (attraction and development) of fibroblast stem cells, and scar formation. It also generates oxidative stress. Recovery from injury is accelerated by highdose antioxidants daily, including vitamin C (3,000mg intravenous [IV]), vitamin E (3,000IU oral), and selenium (200mcg intravenous). These prevent inflammation in the microcirculation level (capillaries), improve the overall health of the recovering patient, and reduce mortality and the length of hospital stays.[323] In burn patients, vitamin C reduces the body's need for fluids and increases urine output, both of which benefit recovery.[324]

The health of critically ill surgery patients in intensive care was greatly improved by vitamin C (3,000mg IV) and vitamin E (3,000IU oral), reducing their rate of multiple organ failure by 57 percent, and shortening their stay in the intensive care unit.[325] The recovery from critical illness and injury is accelerated by omega-3 fatty acids, vitamin C, zinc, and selenium.[326] These effects are thought to be due to the reduction in oxidative stress and inflammation.

Eye surgery is similar to other types of surgery in that it causes oxidative stress, inflammation, and an immune response. After introcular eye surgery, the makeup of the aqueous humor changes. In normal aqueous, the vitamin C level is concentrated by the ciliary epithelia by up to a factor of twenty-five, but typically after surgery this is greatly reduced,[327] implying increased oxidative stress. The vitamin C level of the aqueous humor of diurnal animals (active in the day) is higher than for nocturnal animals, suggesting that the high level of vitamin C is helpful in preventing oxidative stress caused by light.[328] After surgery, the tissue heals by constructing scars consisting of collagen. Because vitamin C is required for collagen synthesis and vitamin C in the aqueous humor is lowered after surgery, this suggests that supplements of vitamin C can help recovery from eye surgery as it does in recovery from trauma and other types of surgery. Indeed, vitamin C accelerates collagen synthesis in human fibroblasts, the cells that stitch together the collagen tissue in scars.[329]

Because vitamin E is known to help wound healing and prevent scarring,[330] it is also recommended along with vitamin C for recovery from surgery. A combination of oral vitamin C and amino acids improved the recovery from surgery for corneal ulcers, suggesting that recovery from any type of corneal surgery will be accelerated with vitamin C.[331] Topically applied N-acetylcysteine, a precursor for glutathione, a powerful antioxidant, lowers inflammation after laser surgery on the cornea.[332]

VITAMIN DEFICIENCIES IN EYES OF INFANTS AND CHILDREN

Newborn babies are especially prone to oxidative stress.[333] Their antioxidant systems have not developed fully, and the higher level of oxygen they receive from their lungs tends to increase the level of free radicals in the eye. Moreover, the flow in their retinal blood vessels is not regulated, so the photoreceptors tend to have a high level of oxidative stress.[334] Premature infants were often treated with high levels of oxygen before this was understood.[335] Oxygen therapy tends to cause the vasculature of the premature retina to lag in development. When the therapy is terminated, the normal air and abnormally developed vasculature do not provide enough oxygen, which causes further changes resulting in retinopathy (damage to the retina).[336]

In addition, the newborn eye receives more oxidative stress from light than the adult eye because the lens is clearer and transmits more blue and UV light. This can cause the buildup of lipofuscin early in life, which in turn causes more light-driven oxidative stress. This may tend to predispose the individual, in adult life, to macular degeneration or other diseases caused by oxidative stress. When infants were given supplements of lutein, their level of oxidative stress was lessened,[337] and other antioxidants likely can help prevent the unique susceptibility of infants to eye disease.[338]

Iron is another cause of oxidative stress in the eye that is relevant to infants. It is normally almost absent in mother's milk, which helps to prevent bacterial infections. Normal-term breastfed babies don't require any supplemental iron in their diet for their first nine to twelve months. They can absorb about 1mg per day from their mother's milk, which is sufficient for growth. However, cow's milk contains less absorbable iron, so babies fed on formula can get anemic without supplements of iron, especially in their second six months. The iron added to infant formula is nonheme bound, which can be a risk factor for bacterial infections and can also promote damage from oxidative stress in the eye during early development.[339] Thus, supplementation with antioxidants in early childhood may be helpful in preventing damage to photoreceptors.

The eye requires vitamin A throughout infancy and childhood. Vitamin A deficiency is the leading cause of blindness in children worldwide.[340] The first symptom of a vitamin A deficiency is night blindness, caused by the eye's inability to regenerate visual pigment in the rod photoreceptors. In a more severe deficiency the lining of cells on the outside of the eye, the conjunctiva, becomes dysfunctional and cannot release mucus and fluid to lubricate the eyeball. This can lead to an inflammation of the cornea, which can lead to ulcers and blindness if severe. These symptoms can be readily reversed if vitamin A deficiency is alleviated with adequate doses. A typical dose is 25IU of vitamin A per pound per day; for instance, 500IU for a twenty-pound child, or the equivalent seven-fold dose once a week. However, once the cornea is damaged by ulceration, the damage is difficult to reverse.[341] Mothers who have sufficient vitamin A in their diet will also tend to have sufficient vitamin A in their breast milk. However, a vitamin-A deficiency in the mother will also cause a deficiency and disease in the infant.[342] In developed countries, infant formula and many breakfast foods are supplemented with vitamin A, so severe vitamin-A deficiencies are rare in these countries.

The inclusion of DHA (an omega-3 fatty acid) in infant formula is important for proper eye development and function. It is found in mother's milk, especially if the mother eats an adequate quantity of oily fish. Traditionally infant formula contained little EPA or DHA, but formula is supplemented with DHA today because it helps the infant's photoreceptors to function. In some studies, no difference was found in eye function between mother's milk and formula supplemented with DHA, but in these studies the DHA content of the mother's milk was low.[343] Therefore, mothers breast-feeding their infants should take care to eat oily fish (such as sardines and salmon) or take fish and flaxseed oil supplements.

CHAPTER 8

EATING RIGHT TO PREVENT EYE DISEASE

This chapter summarizes how vitamin and nutrient supplements can prevent or slow the progression of eye disease. Many age-related eye diseases have a common set of origins, and taking nutritional supplements and eating an excellent diet will reduce your risk of developing them.

If you are interested in continuing your research on preventing eye disease through nutrition and supplementation, a good next step can be found in a series of three review articles by Head and Gaby in *Alternative Medicine Review.* These informative overviews offer compelling evidence about how nutrient supplements can help to prevent ocular diseases when given in the proper dose, method of administration, and length of treatment.[344] You can find the full text of these articles available for free on the Internet.

FINDING THE BALANCE BETWEEN DIET AND SUPPLEMENTS

For vitamins and nutrients to be effective in helping to prevent and treat disease, the dose is extremely important. The reason, as explained in Chapter 1, is that each body has specific needs in its metabolism and maintenance and these needs are set by an individual's genetics, lifestyle, and diet.[345] Although vitamins were thought only necessary in a specific small dose early in the 20th century, today our knowledge has extended the original idea. We now know that the minimum daily requirement is just that-a minimum-for many vitamins and nutrients, and for most people it should not be considered sufficient. Pauling explained that because vitamins are cofactors in many enzyme reactions in our metabolism, the availability of an extra amount of many vitamins helps the necessary metabolic reactions proceed more fully.[346] The studies on eye diseases reviewed in the last several chapters have reiterated this principle, and show that high doses of vitamins and nutrients can make a difference in preventing and treating eye disease. But because each person's requirement for vitamins and nutrients is different, it is important for each individual to understand their unique nutritional requirements.

We know from thousands of laboratory and clinical studies that excellent nutrition can help prevent eye disease. This knowledge raises the question of what doses of nutrients an individual should take, how much of each nutrient is supplied by an excellent diet, and how much should be taken as a supplement. Nutritional supplements are helpful to make sure your body is getting enough nutrition, but they should not be used as a panacea or to transform a bad diet into a good one. Instead, they should be a part of a well-balanced diet, with plenty of fresh fruits and vegetables, especially green leafy vegetables that contain lutein and zeaxanthin. For some, this type of excellent diet may seem adequate, but supplements are recommended for many people by their doctors and nutritionists. The reason, very simply, is that processed food is a large part of most people's daily diet. Any source of calories that is processed or refined will generally not contain the essential nutrients found in the original foods. For this reason, supplements are an acceptable way to assure getting enough vitamins and nutrients for many people, although they cannot take the place of a good diet.

High blood sugar is important to avoid for many eye diseases. Even if you are not diabetic, you can prevent damage from high levels of blood sugar with a low-glycemic-index diet, in which you eat foods that minimize the quick release of sugar into the bloodstream. For example, whole-grain cereals such as quinoa, whole wheat, and oats, without much added sugar, are preferable over other types of sugary and starchy foods such as cake, taro, rice, and refined sugar. With this type of healthy eating, you can lower your blood sugar levels and reduce your risk of the oxidative damage that worsen most eye diseases.

Our ancestors, the early primates, ate a lot of fresh food such as berries, leaves, and fruits. This diet gave them a generous portion of the essential nutrients. It has been estimated that great apes and humans eating lots of wild vegetable foods get 2,000–3,000 milligrams (mg) per day of vitamin C,[347] and also high levels of vitamin A (carotene), and other essential nutrients such as magnesium and calcium. These nutrients can help prevent disease. Here are some ideas on ways to incorporate into your diet raw vegetables that will help to prevent and reverse eye disease.

To maximize your nutrition, a good plan is to eliminate as much refined sugar, flour, and oils as possible. That means no cookies, crackers, cake, pastries, no sweetened granola, no candy, minimal use of salad oil and cooking oils, and minimal fatty foods. It also means no white or "wheat" rolls or bread, that invariably contain enriched flour. Further, it means no pasta made from refined flour that has had its bran and germ removed. Pasta made from semolina, which is a coarse grind of the starchy part of the wheat kernel, is stripped of the bran and germ, so it lacks most of the grain's original vitamins and nutrients such as magnesium. Whole-wheat pasta is OK. Whole-grain flour is preferable, but only if it is fresh, without rancidity, and is truly whole grain. Enriched flour has been processed, and though some B vitamins have been added, it is missing most of the essential trace elements and nutrients such as magnesium that are contained in whole-wheat flour. If you want something sweet, use unrefined (dark brown) sugar, honey, or maple syrup, but only sparingly. These contain some trace elements, but they still are mostly sugar, so you should minimize your use of them. Overall, the effect of this diet is to remove a large excess source of empty calories.

If you don't eat cookies, crackers, most breads, pastries, and pastas, and foods containing a lot of fat and cholesterol, you'll need to fill up on an alternate source of calories. Although meat contains good quantities of essential nutrients, it contains a lot of calories and is often consumed in excess. The best idea is to substitute vegetables, fruits, and nuts. Raw vegetables such as carrots, celery, red and green peppers, and tomatoes are chock-full of nutrients, and virtually any type of fruit such as apples, pears, oranges, bananas, melons, and berries are excellent. Sprouts are excellent. Of course, one of the best categories of vegetables are green leafy vegetables (collards, kale, cabbage, Brussels sprouts, broccoli, spinach, Chinese cabbage, Swiss chard, and such), because they contain almost all the nutrients you need. Nuts and seeds such as almonds, peanuts, pistachios, walnuts, and sunflower and pumpkin seeds contain generous amounts of nutrients but also many calories. Walnuts contain less protein than some other nuts, but are high in ALA, the essential omega-3 fatty acid. You can learn more about what is included in the low-glycemic-index diet by reading up on the science of food and nutrition.[348] If you eat a good quantity of fresh vegetables you can get the extra calories you've sacrificed by forgoing refined foods.

At the same time you'll obtain a lot of vitamins and nutrients.

Another essential part of obtaining adequate nutrients is to chew your food thoroughly.[349] The reason is that digestive enzymes and stomach acid, which are responsible for breaking down food for digestion, can only do their job if the particles of food are small. This is especially important for nuts and raw vegetables. Try to chew nuts long enough to reduce them to a very small size. I buy smooth nut butters, not chunky, for the same reason-they are more digestible. Thorough chewing mixes food particles with saliva, which contains enzymes that help digest starches, such as those found in pasta, potatoes, and bread.

Suggestions for Eye Health: Sprouts and Green Smoothies

Sprouts make an excellent meal, or for beginners, an excellent side dish. They are relatively inexpensive, and very easy to prepare and chew.[350] Several types of sprouts are commonly available, and alfalfa and bean seeds are often sprouted and eaten raw.

Another excellent health food relevant to treatment of eye disease is the green smoothie. This is a very enjoyable way to get lots of excellent nutrition into your diet without much effort.[351]

Sprouting Seeds

The basic recipe for sprouting seeds is simple. Go to the supermarket or health food store and buy the dry seeds. You can sprout alfalfa, wheat, buckwheat, clover, many types of beans and lentils, quinoa, and for a zippy flavor, radishes. Make sure that the seeds are meant for eating and not sowing in the soil, to avoid any chemical treatments. Pour two to three layers of the seeds into a waterproof container such as a flat-bottomed plastic food storage container or glass jar. Cover them with water overnight (six to eight hours) and drain them the next morning. The seeds should be fresh, and the water should be unchlorinated. You can remove chlorine from your tap water with a purifying carbon filter. The seeds will germinate and start to sprout in a day or so.

Each day, morning and night, add enough water to cover the seeds. Swirl them gently in the water to rinse them well, and drain them, preferably twice. This is important for two reasons: it provides water for the sprouts to grow, and it helps to wash out any bacteria that have appeared. Once the seeds have sprouted, you can eat them right away. You can also continue to wash and drain them twice a day while they grow. Once their rootlets have grown several millimeters long you can store them in the refrigerator for a few days. In the summer warmth, the sprouts will grow faster and will be ready in one or two days. It will take a little longer in the winter, depending on the temperature.

Sprouts are remarkable! As explained in Chapter 1, they can contribute to a slowing or reversal of eye disease. They contain many essential vitamins, minerals, omega-3 fatty acids, and protein. You can buy them already sprouted at a local health food store if you don't want to sprout them yourself. They're a complete meal!

Green Smoothies

Green smoothies are not only enjoyable-they provide superior nutrition and are easy to make. You simply put your favorite dark green leafy vegetables, such as spinach, collards, kale, broccoli, arugula, mustard greens, Swiss chard, dandelions, romaine lettuce, or similar vegetables into a blender with some liquid, and blend to a fine consistency that you can drink. Collard or kale greens are an excellent choice, for they are as nutritious as spinach and generally less expensive. Of course, collards are also excellent when cooked. A favorite dish of mine is chopped collards and onions, steamed for a few minutes. But a green smoothie that includes raw collards can be even more nutritious and tasty.

Collards, kale, and other dark green leafy vegetables in the same species *brassica oleracea* (broccoli, Brussels sprouts, cabbage) are terrific for nutrition. They contain a whole range of healthy nutrients including vitamin A, many of the B vitamins including folate, vitamin C, vitamin E, vitamin K, lutein and zeaxanthin, magnesium, protein, and many others.[352] This combination of nutrients is thought to be especially good for preventing age-related eye diseases, such as macular degeneration, retinitis pigmentosa, and glaucoma. For example, a generous helping of collards at least once a week may reduce your risk of glaucoma by 50 percent or more.[353] Although the amount of protein in a cup of collards (5 grams) doesn't seem like a lot, you'll get enough protein and also a robust amount of the other beneficial vitamins and nutrients if you eat enough to satisfy hunger.

Collards are easy to grow in your backyard garden. They can be started in early spring and will grow through the summer season until the first frost. They are very inexpensive at the supermarket, but I prefer to grow my own because that way I know they are clean and without pesticides. For a one-quart smoothie you can blend three or four big collard leaves. For some spicy zip, it's great to add a little arugula or mustard greens (which are also very easy to grow). Although one to two cups of water is good for a quart blender, I prefer to use juice such as orange or cranberry juice, unfiltered natural cider, mixed vegetable juice, or pomegranate juice. These add extra nutrients as well as a little sweetness to the smoothie that makes it more palatable for many people. For an extra boost you can add other ingredients, such as nutritional or brewer's yeast or nuts; for example, peanuts, almonds, or walnuts.

To make the smoothie, add the liquid first and add the collard or kale leaves one at a time. After you add each leaf, replace the blender top and turn the blender on for a few seconds. Stop the blender and add another leaf, and repeat the process. Keep the blender on for another minute or so after you've blended in several leaves. Then turn it off and enjoy a very green-tasting beverage.

For a sweeter green smoothie, for example for dessert, add an extra cup of fruit such as apples, pears, peaches, or blueberries to your two cups of dark green leafy vegetables. There's no limit to ideas about what ingredients to combine. Green smoothies will give you lots of vitamin A, lutein and zeaxanthin, vitamin C, calcium, magnesium, and a generous amount of other essential nutrients like omega-3 fatty acids and protein.

Like sprouts, smoothies are a healthy, delicious, complete meal!

Eating Right All Day

Along with fresh vegetables and fruits, your daily meals can benefit from whole-grain products. At breakfast, a good way to start the day is with whole-grain wheat or oats, typically eaten with dairy products such as milk or yogurt. Rolled one-minute or five-minute oats are a bargain and need not be cooked, because the steam-heated rolling process makes them easily digestible without additional cooking when they are chewed properly. Wheat germ or brewer's yeast added to oats provides additional nutrition. Avoid commercial breakfast cereal, even when it is fortified with vitamins, because it generally contains processed flour with little magnesium and it costs much more. Lunch might include wholegrain bread along with nuts or nut butter, or a serving of fish, chicken, or a little meat, and fresh vegetables such as salad greens, carrots, tomatoes, and fruit. Dinner might include a large serving of fresh raw vegetables such as sprouts, spinach, lettuce, arugula, carrots, green or red peppers, celery, and tomatoes, with whole-grain bread or pasta, along with beans, fish, or a little meat, and generous servings of cooked fresh or frozen vegetables such as green beans, potatoes, squash, beets, broccoli, and cabbage. Yogurt, sparingly sweetened, and fresh fruit provide excellent nutrition for dessert.

Several times a week you should have a good-sized serving of leafy green vegetables such as kale; collards; cabbage; Brussels sprouts; spinach; and beet, turnip, or mustard greens, for vitamins A, B, K, and carotenoids. A serving of mixed seeds and nuts without salt, including sunflower seeds, pumpkin seeds, pistachios, almonds, and walnuts will provide an assortment of helpful oils and nutrients. A healthy dessert might include fruit and yogurt. You can combine many of these items into a green smoothie, which will help you digest them. If you eat mostly whole grains, vegetables, nuts, and fruits, you'll naturally get enough potassium and magnesium, and if you include several servings of yogurt or other dairy products you'll get enough calcium. Avoid processed food such as fast food, soups, frozen dinners, crackers, cookies, or cake. Compared to fresh vegetables, processed foods generally contain more calories, more salt (sodium), and fewer nutrients, and they cost more.

But what about vitamins?

RATIONALE FOR SUPPLEMENTS

If you switch to eating a better diet, you may find yourself feeling feeling healthier, with more energy. Your eyes and the rest of the body will be more resistant to disease. But many people find that they have difficulty eliminating all refined foods from their diet. Occasional refined foods will generally not cause much of a problem if they do not represent a large proportion of your daily calories, because you'll still be filling up on other healthy foods. A good rule is to find out what nutrients are missing in the refined food you eat, and then obtain the the missing nutrients from some other source. For example, when I go to a party and am served cake, I'll enjoy eating it but will make a mental note about how many calories the serving contained. Later I'll substitute a more nutrient-containing food. To find out what nutrients are in common foods, you can look up the nutritional content online.[354] This checking may appeal to some people, but many have not found the time to learn the details of all the nutrients in the foods they eat. This is the rationale behind taking nutrient supplements. Instead of trying to total up all the vitamins and minerals in the refined and unrefined foods you eat, you can eat a good diet with lots of fruits and vegetables, and then simply take extra supplements to make sure that you are getting enough vitamins and minerals.

How to Resolve Contradictions about Doses

Nutrition is a complex topic, and much about the effect of nutrition on eye diseases remains to be discovered. While many observational studies have shown a benefit of vitamins A, B, C, and E on eye disease, in recent years some randomized controlled trials (RCTs) designed to test the benefit of these nutrients have not shown statistically significant health benefits.[355] Some of the conditions of the large studies may seem confusing. For example, it is apparent that an RCT cannot give a meaningful test of a vitamin treatment if the treatment is limited to too low or too high a dose, even when the RCT attempts to achieve statistical significance by averaging random fluctuation over a sufficiently large population.

One of the main factors in the decision about dosage in health studies is the possibility that the nutrients when given in large doses might cause harm. Thus, quite often the doses given are small. Although there is a high level that can cause harm for every nutrient, there are only a few nutrients, such as vitamin A, iron and selenium, for which this is a big concern, and these are well-known although not widely understood. It is easy to avoid toxic doses of vitamins and minerals as long as one takes a few simple precautions. However, conservatism seems to be widespread in the motivation to avoid overdoses. A propensity to eat what our parents and culture taught us appears to be a feature of the brain, even when there is reliable new evidence showing the benefits of new choices. Thus tradition appears to be one of the factors in the selection of dose and the scientific questions asked by health studies.

This situation may seem difficult to sort out, even to the interested health-conscious person. One might imagine that apparently contradictory conclusions from different studies, for example, an observational study and an RCT, represent a failure of science. It might seem that either the observational study or the RCT were inherently flawed.[356] But it is entirely reasonable that the conclusions of both are correct and thus without conflict, because their scientific questions were different or they were susceptible to different problems. When an observational study on a specific at-risk group shows a benefit of supplements and is backed up by a likely mechanism such as preventing oxidative stress, a negative result in an RCT does not trump the positive result in the observational study.[357] The reason is that RCTs, like observational studies, can be confounded by bias factors, such as the complexities of diet, daily habits such as smoking, and related physiological and disease states. For example, some participants in RCTs may be at risk because they have early indications of disease. If they take supplements as a remedy, this may confuse the conclusions of the study. Alternately, participants who take supplements may be health-conscious individuals who have no indications of disease. Both of these possibilities introduce bias into a health study about the benefits of supplements, which can confound the conclusions of the study.[358]

Because of this, it seems likely that the generally mixed results from RCTs testing the benefits of antioxidants already known to be helpful for prevention of eye disease are often a direct consequence of the low doses given.[359] For example, the amount of vitamin C typically taken in RCTs, typically 500mg or less, would not be expected to show a large effect, and the effects of low supplement levels on eye diseases are likely to be confounded by differences in diet correlated with other risk factors.[360] Further, many RCTs of antioxidants on eye diseases have collected only short-term data, less than twelve months, on antioxidant intake. Because oxidative damage in the eye is age-related, antioxidants are more likely to be beneficial when taken at high doses over several decades.

There also is concern in the scientific literature about risks of taking supplements of high levels of essential nutrients, but much of this concern appears to be misplaced. Some is only applicable to individuals with rare genetic conditions that require special care about supplemental doses of some essential nutrients, so if you have special conditions you should consult with a nutrition-aware medical professional. The levels of nutrients recommended below are very safe for most people.

Smoking

n any discussion of what to eat for optimal health, it is appropriate to consider what substances not to take into the body. Number one is smoke, which is an important risk factor for cardiovascular disease, lung diseases including cancer, and also for eye disease.[361] Thousands of toxic chemicals enter the body from smoking. They are harmful in the short term and in the long term.[362] Each puff of cigarette smoke gives approximately 1017 oxidant molecules that can damage the retina and retinal pigment epithelium (RPE).[363] The more smoke someone inhales, the worse the effects become. Smoking increases the risk of cataract by almost a factor of three.[364] The reason is likely that smoking causes oxidative stress on the entire body, including the blood and eye tissues. The oxidative stress greatly reduces the amount of vitamin C and vitamin E in the bloodstream.[365] Smokers also tend to have higher levels of lead and cadmium in their body and eye tissues. These toxic metal ions are a risk factor for cataracts, at least in part because they to lower the level of vitamins C and E in the bloodstream.[366]

Supplements of antioxidants such as vitamins C and E can help counteract some of the toxic effects.[367]

Smoking is one of most important risk factors for age-related macular degeneration (AMD). The reason is likely that smoking causes oxidative damage throughout the tissues of the eye.[368] Studies of the effects of smoking on AMD have shown a twofold increased risk of AMD, and if you have certain genetic mutations, smoking can increase your risk for AMD up to thirtyfold.[369] Inhaling any kind of smoke, including secondhand cigarette or cigar smoke, is almost as bad as active smoking. Some of the toxins present in cigarette smoke are known to induce cell death in the RPE,[370] which is thought to be directly linked to initiation of AMD.[371] The toxins in smoke also cause the eye to express vascular endothelial growth factor (VEGF), which is thought to be involved in initiating wet AMD.[372]

Several studies of the effects of vitamins have shown that smoking reduces or counteracts the helpful effects of vitamin and nutrient supplements. For example, as mentioned above, several RCTs showed that in those who take beta-carotene, smoking reversed its beneficial effect and increased the risk of lung cancer. The reason for the interaction between smoking and beta-carotene is currently unknown, but it appears to be specific to those taking beta-carotene supplements who smoke. When beta-carotene is given together with vitamin C and vitamin E, there is no increase in risk for smokers, and beta-carotene given to nonsmokers does not increase the risk.[373]

A similar finding has been reported about vitamin E. It appears from some RCTs that smoking can reverse the beneficial effect of vitamin E in older people who take this supplement, increasing the risk of complications like pneumonia.[374] The effect of smoking on the beneficial effect of vitamin E is mitigated by adequate vitamin C and, of course, by reducing the amount of smoking.[375] Similarly, in some RCTs, smoking apparently reverses the benefits of folate and vitamin B_{12}.[376] In all of these studies, the beneficial effects of the nutrient supplement was already established. B eta-carotene is helpful for the eye because it can supply vitamin A in a form that is nontoxic in large doses. Vitamin E, taken along with other antioxidants, can help prevent many age-related diseases, including cardiovascular disease, cancer, and eye diseases. When reading these studies one might imagine that good advice for smokers would be to avoid taking vitamin and nutrient supplements. But in fact the opposite is true. Better advice appears to be to stop smoking immediately. You'll derive a tremendous benefit if you stop smoking, eat a healthy diet, and take supplements of vitamins and nutrients.

SUPPLEMENT DOSES

A good plan for many people is to start by taking a multivitamin and mineral tablet. Multivitamin tablets are commonly available that contain a variety of vitamins in specific ratios known to be beneficial. "Health" or "mega" multivitamin tablets contain higher levels of vitamins and generally contain more trace elements and helpful nutrients. You also may want to supplement with additional amounts of selected nutrients that are not provided in the multivitamin tablet.

Vitamin A

To keep your photoreceptors healthy, vitamin A (retinol) is essential. Vitamin A is also utilized as an important growth factor in a partially metabolized form (retinoic acid) by tissues throughout the body, including the epithelial cells of arteries and the skin. Along with these specific functions for the eye, tissues, and skin, vitamin A is an important antioxidant. A common dose of vitamin A is 5,000-10,000 international units (IU) per day, depending on your body weight (25-50IU per pound per day). Because many multivitamin tablets contain 5,000-10,000IU, one tablet daily will give you an adequate dose. Vitamin A is actively taken up by the liver, which can store enough for several months, regulating the blood level to be relatively constant. Because it is fat-soluble, its level in the body takes several months to rise or fall. The consequence of this is that you must take a daily dose for several months to get a benefit. However, if you drink alcohol, your requirement of vitamin A is increased.

Concerns about Vitamin A

There are several concerns about vitamin A. First, it can be toxic if taken at too high a dose, but the toxicity is not always apparent right away. With a high daily dose, toxic effects can appear with a delay of six months or more. Although a dose of 5,000-10,000IU per day is considered safe for most people,[377] those with special circumstances such as pregnancy or problems like kidney disease should be aware of its potential toxicity. Sometimes doses of 25,000IU are given under medical supervision to treat a specific problem, but it is important not to take this dose for too long or a toxic level could result. Also, those eating liver should keep track of their total ingestion of vitamin A, for liver can contain 100,000IU in a four-ounce portion. And be wary about eating polar bear liver, for even a small portion contains enough vitamin A to produce immediate toxicity.[378]

You can avoid the potential toxicity of vitamin A by substituting beta-carotene, which is nontoxic and can be converted to vitamin A when needed by the body.[379] If you eat a lot of green or orange vegetables, you needn't worry about getting too much extra vitamin A, because only the amount of beta-carotene the body needs is converted to the active form of vitamin A. The beta-carotene in supplements is about 50 percent as effective as vitamin A, and most dietary sources of beta-carotene are about 10 percent as effective. The IU of vitamin A is 0.3 micrograms (mcg) of retinol.[380] So the recommended daily amount (3,000IU) is equivalent to 900mcg of vitamin A, about 2mg of beta-carotene in supplements, or about 10mg of dietary beta-carotene.

There have also been concerns reported about high levels of supplementary beta-carotene. It can help to prevent eye disease, and in observational studies the consumption of vegetables and higher blood levels of beta-carotene have been shown to reduce risk for lung cancer.[381] However, when this hypothesis was tested in several interventional studies, they showed that beta-carotene increased the risk of lung cancer in smokers.[382] The reason is currently unknown, but appears to be specific to smokers given only beta-carotene, because there is no increase in risk when beta-carotene is given together with vitamin C and vitamin E,[383] and beta-carotene alone does not increase the risk to nonsmokers. One hypothesis suggests that the oxygen-rich environment of the lung causes special problems for tissue damaged by smoke. Many medical researchers have therefore argued against supplementation with beta-carotene. However, the studies showing the effect were done on smokers, who were at a very high risk of cancer before they were included in the trial. Because beta-carotene has been shown to be helpful in preventing eye disease, it seems wise to continue to supplement with it at an adequate level, along with other supplements and a healthy diet, and to stop smoking.

The best advice regarding vitamin A supplementation appears to be: take 5,000–10,000IU per day, along with other nutrients, in a diet that includes green vegetables such as spinach, kale, collards, broccoli, or orange vegetables like carrots, sweet potatoes, and pumpkin. These vegetables contain beta-carotene, which is converted to vitamin A by the body. Eggs, whole-milk products, and fish liver oils are excellent sources. And, of course, liver is a rich source of vitamin A, but keep track of your intake to avoid toxicity. If you eat one good-sized carrot per day, you'll get about 10mg of beta-carotene,[384] which is equivalent to about 3,000IU of vitamin A. If you eat too many carrots, you may find your skin turning orange-yellowish, but this is not harmful-just reduce your carrot intake.

The Vitamin Bs

The B vitamins are important nutrients essential for maintenance and energy in the body's metabolic reactions. They are usually taken together, because they are required by the body's metabolism in specific ratios. They are water-soluble and you need to take daily doses of several of them. Thiamine, riboflavin, and niacin (vitamins B_1, B_2, and B_3) are often included in multivitamin tablets because they have little risk and potentially a big benefit from preventing a deficiency. Many multivitamin tablets include relatively low amounts (1–20mg), but mega multivitamin tablets often supply much higher amounts (50–100mg), which are safe. A deficiency of the B vitamins leads to loss of nerve and brain function, memory loss, irritability, and depression.[385] Riboflavin (50mg per day) is an antioxidant and is needed for a variety of metabolic reactions, including within the red blood cells.

Niacin (50–2,000mg per day, divided doses) is helpful in dilating blood vessels, which may be important in the eye for preventing retinal disease associated with lack of nutrition, such as retinitis pigmentosa. One concern when taking niacin is that in rare cases, for example, in less than 1 percent of people taking high doses (3,000mg per day) to lower cholesterol, niacin can cause problems in the eye, such as cystoid macular edema. These problems are unrelated to leakage from blood vessels in diabetic retinopathy, because they are reversible. When those who develop this problem discontinue niacin or reduce the dose below a critical threshold, for example, 1,000mg per day, the cystoid maculopathy typically goes away within a few weeks. If you note any visual problems when taking niacin, especially in reading, which utilizes the macula, your opthalmologist can check for this problem and may recommend reducing your niacin dose.[386] When first taking niacin, start with a small dose (25-50mg, the amount in many multivitamins) and then slowly increase the dose over several days. If you take too much at once, you may feel a warmth and redness on your skin, which is known as a "niacin flush." This is usually considered harmless and typically disappears in thirty to sixty minutes. Gradually over several weeks you can slowly increase the daily dose, up to 1,000mg or more, without getting a flush. Niacin at this level can also help to increase high-density lipoprotein (HDL) and lower your cholesterol, which keeps your cardiovascular system healthy and helps to prevent heart disease. Although niacin can temporarily increase blood pressure, this can be largely prevented by taking it with vitamins C, D, and E, and magnesium. An alternate form of niacin, called niacinamide or nicotinamide, doesn't cause flushing, but it seems best to avoid taking this form of B_3. It does not lower cholesterol and at high doses (greater than 3,000mg per day) has been reported to cause liver damage.

Like most of the B vitamins, vitamin B_5(pantothenate, 50mg per day) is important for the metabolic reactions of all the tissues. Vitamin B_5 is necessary for healing of wounds and helps epithelial tissues, such as the surface of the cornea and the conjunctiva, to heal.[387] It is transported into epithelial cells along with biotin and lipoic acid, implying that the tissues require these nutrients together.[388] Biotin (vitamin B_7) is an essential cofactor in the metabolic pathways of cells,[389] and its deficiency can cause severe illness including cancer.[390] It is so essential for life that egg white contains avidin, a biotin-binding protein that prevents bacteria invading the egg from utilizing biotin for growth. Thus, eating raw egg white tends to cause a biotin deficiency unless a good source of biotin is available, such as meat or a multivitamin supplement. Egg white also contains several other antibacterial and antiviral substances that are denatured when the egg is cooked.[391]

Vitamins B_6 (pyridoxine, 50mg per day), B_9 (folate, 2.5mg per day), and B_{12} (cyanocobalamin, 1mg per day) were shown to be helpful in preventing age-related macular degeneration (AMD).[392] These levels are higher than contained in a typical multivitamin tablet, but they are thought to be safe and without serious side effects.

Vitamin B_{12} and folate are related, and both are very important for every cell in the body for synthesis of DNA and in energy production. They are essential for tissues of the brain and retina. A vitamin-B_{12} deficiency is common among vegetarians, and a good solution for many is a vitamin B_{12} supplement. The body absorbs vitamin B_{12} with a special protein-binding factor and a dedicated transporter that captures the minute quantities available in food. Thus, a deficiency of vitamin B_{12} can also reflect a problem with this special uptake system.[393] A standard blood test is available to find out if you have an adequate intake and absorption of folate and vitamin B_{12}. Good sources of folate are the green leafy vegetables (from which the name "folate" derives), seeds, and beans and legumes. Vitamin B_{12} is not made by plants or animals, but is made by certain types of bacteria. Good sources are shellfish, liver, sardines, and salmon, and meat contains a little. Supplementary tablets of vitamin B_{12} (cyanocobalamin, methylcobalamin) are widely available containing 1,000 micrograms (1mg), a tiny amount, but hundreds of times greater than the body's daily requirement. There appears to be little risk in taking this excessive amount, but generally a supplement only needs to be taken when a blood test indicates a deficiency. The body can store enough vitamin B_{12} in the liver for several years, so if you aren't getting enough in your diet, you may not notice any problem immediately. Likewise, if you eat liver for several meals you may get enough vitamin B_{12} to last your body several months.

You may notice some side effects when taking multivitamin supplements that contain B vitamins. Riboflavin (vitamin B_2) is orange-yellowish in color so will color your urine. This is usually harmless. There are of course other symptoms that can be signaled by colored urine, but if you notice bright-yellow urine after taking a tablet with vitamin B_{21} this is normal. And as mentioned above, niacin (vitamin B_3) can cause a temporary red flush on the skin that is usually harmless.

Vitamin C

Vitamin C (ascorbate) is a powerful antioxidant and an important water-soluble vitamin necessary for the body. It is essential for many important biochemical reactions, including synthesis of collagen that holds the body together. It can reduce intraocular pressure, and so is an effective way to prevent and treat glaucoma.[394] It strengthens arteries, prevents inflammation, and lowers the risk of cardiovascular disease and heart failure,[395] which is extremely helpful in preventing many eye diseases. Although concern has often been voiced about high doses of vitamin C, it is nontoxic and nonimmunogenic,[396] sc the doses suggested in this book are safe for most people.

Vitamin C in its oxidized form, dehydroascorbate, is preferentially taken up by red blood cells where it can be reduced back to ascorbate to continue its antioxidant and enzyme cofactor functions.[397] This happens only in primates, guinea pigs, and fruit-eating bats, that is, animals that cannot make their own ascorbate. Although we can survive in the short term without the large quantities that other animal continually make, high doses can help us stay in optimal health.[398] Also note that a diet high in fat and cholesterol increases the use of vitamin C, and thus lowers the vitamin C levels in the brain,[399] implying that your need for vitamin C increases when you eat a lot of fat. This will directly affect the health of your retina and other eye tissues.

A common misconception is that the amount of vitamin C in many daily multivitamin tablets, 100–200mg, is adequate for most of us. This dose is inadequate for several reasons. A single dose taken in a multivitamin tablet at breakfast will likely be well absorbed, but it cannot maintain a high blood level throughout the day. Vitamin C is needed in much higher amounts, for most people 3,000–10,000mg per day, as explained in Chapter 1. It is important to take vitamin C in divided doses for the highest absorption and utilization. Those of us who are exposed to toxins in the environment need to take special care to get an adequate amount of vitamin C. Many toxins, such as smoke, cause oxidative stress that can worsen eye disease. Smokers have a lower level of vitamin C in their blood, which is directly caused by the oxidative stress of the toxins in smoke. The vitamin C can neutralize the toxins from the smoke but in doing so it becomes oxidized. To remain effective it must be reduced again by red blood cells, or replaced by fresh vitamin C. Any toxin or stress induced by bacterial or viral infection lowers the level of vitamin C in the blood, which in turn lowers the body's protection from any other source of oxidative stress.[400] This is particularly important for the eye, which concentrates vitamin C by twenty-five-fold above the blood level. The eye requires this high concentration of vitamin C to prevent oxidative stress from its high concentration of oxygen and from light. So, if you smoke, you should stop immediately. And take extra vitamin C supplements if you are exposed to any other source of chemical toxin. This will pay off in the long run, preventing oxidative stress in your eyes and throughout your body.

Another common misconception, often heard from medical professionals, is that vitamin C increases the risk of kidney stones because it tends to increase the level of urinary oxalate, a common constituent of kidney stones. Oxalate can precipitate in the urine when a high level of calcium is present, but this can be prevented by increasing the intake of magnesium.[401] High doses of vitamin C can cause the level of oxalate in the urine to increase slightly, which on first thought might suggest an increase in the risk of calcium oxalate kidney stones. But a careful look at the literature reveals no evidence for vitamin C actually causing kidney stones.[402] A high dose of vitamin C, after it has performed its function of reducing oxidative stress in the blood and tissues, tends to increase the level of urinary vitamin C, which does not cause calcium oxalate stones. This is because vitamin C is a diuretic and tends to increase urinary volume. It also binds calcium and prevents it from precipitating,[403] so high doses of vitamin C apparently reduce the tendency to form oxalate stones, even in people prone to them.[404]

There are some known complications of high doses of vitamin C for individuals with impaired kidney function[405] or some rare genetic conditions, for example, those with glucose-6-phosphate dehydrogenase deficiency.[406] However, glucose-6-phosphate deficiency poses little risk for healthy people taking high doses of vitamin C.[407] Overall the risk of serious complications from high vitamin C doses in health) people is very low.[408] Therefore, the concern about high doses of vitamin C causing kidney stones of other problems in healthy individuals seems unwarranted.

A study of a diet specifically designed to reduce hypertension, containing lots of fruits and vegetables, moderate amounts of dairy, and low amounts of animal protein, produced higher urinary levels of calcium, magnesium, potassium, and vitamin C, but also showed reduced kidney stones.[409] One reason for this is that an excellent diet high in fruits and vegetables, especially when it contains large doses of vitamin C, increases urinary volume to prevent stones even when it contains higher levels of oxalate.[410] The intake of vitamin C in this study apparently contributed to the lessened risk.

A common concern about vitamin C is the effect of its acidity on the body. Vitamin C (ascorbic acid) is a weak acid, only slightly stronger than vinegar, but less powerful than citric acid found in lemons. The acidity can cause several problems, but they are easy to deal with. If you chew a vitamin C tablet, the vitamin C in the tablet can stick to your teeth and etch them. To prevent this, purchase a chewable tablet that contains only sodium ascorbate, which is buffered and nonacidic. If you swallow vitamin C tablets without chewing they will not cause any problem with your teeth. Vitamin C can cause an upset stomach in some people because of its acidity when it is taken in high doses, such as 10,000–20,000 m€ per day or more to prevent a viral infection. It is important to note that this acidity, even from a large dose of vitamin C, is less than the normal stomach acidity by many-fold, but the vitamin C tablets ma) take some time to dissolve in the stomach. If you tend to get stomach upset from a large dose of vitamin. C, it is easy to fix using buffered ascorbate. You can purchase buffered ascorbate in the form of sodium, calcium, or magnesium ascorbate. If you take more than your bowel tolerance, you may note a laxative effect and acidity in the stools which can be irritating. However, vitamin C is nontoxic even in huge doses, so the laxative effect is not harmful to the body.[411]

Another aspect of this concern about the acidity of vitamin C is whether taking a large dose could affect the body's acid balance (pH) causing health problems. This is not usually a big concern, because the body can closely regulate its acidity given a healthy diet with lots of fruits and vegetables. Over a short time period, minutes to hours, the autonomic nervous system regulates the rate of breathing. For example, faster breathing removes carbon dioxide from the blood, which reduces its acidity, while slower breathing allows the level of carbon dioxide in the blood to increase, increasing the body's acidity. Over a longer time period, the kidneys take over and can excrete either acid or basic constituents of urine.[412] After vitamin C has done its job of reducing free radicals in the blood and tissues it is readily excreted in the urine as dehydroascorbate (DHAA). And, overall, the body has little difficulty maintaining acid-base balance because vitamin C is a weak acid.

There is also concern that vitamin C increases the uptake of iron, which can be a problem for people who suffer from hemochromatosis, or iron overload disease. The problem is that there is no known physiological pathway for getting rid of extra iron through excretion, so the amount of iron in the body must be regulated in absorption.[413] The body readily absorbs heme iron, the type of iron in red meat, but cannot regulate how much is absorbed. However the absorption of non-heme iron, the type found in vegetables such as spinach, or in supplements, is closely regulated by the level of iron in the body.[414] Vitamin C enhances the absorption of nonheme iron, so vitamin C is sometimes blamed for causing an excess of iron in the body. Those with hemochromatosis may be advised to carefully regulate their intake of red meat and vegetable sources and to avoid vitamin C supplements. However, in normal people, an excess of iron is typically caused by eating too much red meat. Thus you are well-advised to eat a moderate or minimal amount of meat, and to help yourself to generous amounts of beans, lentils, and tomato products. Multivitamin tablets for women typically contain approximately 20mg of iron, and for men, approximately 10mg of iron. But you can also purchase similar multivitamin tablets without iron, You can easily control how much iron you get in your diet by eating vegetable foods that contain iron, along with vitamin C, and with the use of intermittent iron supplementation when needed.

The most common concern about vitamin C appears to be its tendency to cause a laxative effect. When a single large dose or several smaller doses of vitamin C are taken over several hours and the body cannot absorb all of it, the fraction left in the gut tends to attract fluid by osmosis, which can cause gas or a laxative effect. The bowel tolerance for a normal healthy adult can be determined by gradually increasing the dose of vitamin C from 1,000mg per day up to 6,000mg per day or more. The dose should be taken in divided portions throughout the day for the most benefit, because the blood lever rises and falls within a few hours. A low dose of vitamin C will be well below the body's need. As the dose is increased it eventually will go beyond the body's need, and will tend to attract moisture into the gut and cause the laxative effect. When this happens, the dose should be reduced, typically by 20 to 5C percent, until the laxative effect abates. This establishes the bowel tolerance.[415]

To put this in perspective, it is important to understand that vitamin C is selectively taken up by the gut according to the body's need. During an ordinary day, a healthy person may only require a relatively small dose, in the range of 2,000–10,000mg (15–50mg per pound per day). For many people, a dose o 1,000-2,000mg at each meal is well tolerated. But with a severe viral infection or stress, the body car take up vitamin C at a much higher rate, so that 1,000-3,000mg every fifteen minutes is within bowel tolerance.[416] But if this same mega dose is taken when the stress is not present, the gut will not fully absorb it. With experience, one learns to discern the level of stress and to adjust the dose to the body's requirements.

Recently a new form of vitamin C has become available, packaged inside nanoscale phospholipid spheres, called liposomes, much like a cell membrane preserves its contents. The liposomes protect the vitamin C from oxidation and are absorbed by the stomach more readily than straight vitamin C. Liposomal vitamin C is supposed to be five-to tenfold more efficacious in raising the blood level than straight vitamin C. Therefore, a 1,000mg packet of liposomal vitamin C is equivalent to taking 5–10 grams of vitamin C tablets. Liposomal vitamin C is more expensive than vitamin C tablets, but it may be worth the extra cost. The phospholipids in the nanospheres are good for your health because they are used in cell membranes throughout the body.

Vitamin D

In recent years, research on vitamin D has shown it has important roles everywhere in the body. When it was first discovered, it was thought to be essential only for preventing bone problems in children who didn't get much sunlight. Vitamin D is now known to be important for calcium utilization, proper function of the immune system, reducing inflammation, and to prevent many types of disease such as cancer and heart disease.[417] Vitamin D is produced by exposure of the skin to direct sunlight, and is found in only a few unprocessed foods such as oily fish. It is now thought that every cell in the body has vitamin D receptors, which serve to regulate the function of all cells and tissues. Thus, vitamin D is a powerful hormone for tissues throughout the body, including the eye. Vitamin D is relatively easy to get from fortified foods, and it is also safe to take in supplement form. Because a recent study has shown that vitamin D can help to prevent AMD, it is a safe, easy, and effective way to enhance your eye health.[418]

Although it's easy to get an adequate level of vitamin D in the summer when the sun is high in the sky, the amount of sunlight required to give a daily dose varies widely.[419] The reason is that short wavelength UV light (UVB), which is uniquely able to generate vitamin D in your skin, is only available from direct exposure to sunlight when the sun is 45 degrees or more above the horizon. Window glass absorbs almost all the UVB in sunlight, so sitting behind a window won't give you any vitamin D, and exposure to the sun in the early morning, late afternoon, or anytime in the winter in the lower forty-eight states, will provide almost none. Even if you get a little tan from winter sunlight you won't be getting much vitamin D, unless the sun is above 45 degrees from the horizon. Moreover, the effective dose of vitamin D you get also depends on the color of your skin. People with light skin can get enough vitamin D (10,000IU) wearing shorts and a short-sleeve shirt in about fifteen minutes from exposure to midday summer sunlight. However, if your skin is dark, it may take ninety minutes or more to get the same dose. So, for office workers who are inside most of the day, a vitamin D supplement is an excellent way to get your dose. Because vitamin D is fat-soluble, its absorption depends to some extent on the amount of fat you eat. The level of vitamin D in the body builds up and falls slowly, so you need to take a daily dose for several months before the level in the body gets to its eventual equilibrium. This also means that you don't need to take vitamin D every day. If you get a larger dose on the weekends, your body will store the extra vitamin D for use over the next week.

Interestingly, and highlighting the importance of vitamin D for health, it is currently thought that vitamin D is responsible for the light skin color of humans living away from the equator.[420] When. modern humans evolved in Africa, 50,000 to 100,000 years ago, their skin color was dark like the skin to many Africans today. But as people migrated north out of Africa their ability to generate vitamin D from sunlight was compromised, because at high latitudes the amount of UVB available from sunlight is greatly reduced.[421] Some of their descendants developed lighter skin color due to random genetic mutations.

Because they generated more vitamin D in their skin, and because of the importance of vitamin D to health, these lighter-skinned descendants survived better in northern Europe and Asia. This process of natural selection can change human skin color from dark to light, or from light to dark in a period of 50 to 100 generations. The evolutionary force selecting skin color to be dark near the equator is due to the fact exposure to bright sunlight degrades folate (vitamin B_9) in the blood underneath the skin. Because a folate deficiency in a mother causes spina bifida, which is usually fatal, in the unborn child, there was a tremendous evolutionary pressure toward dark skin in Africa where sunlight contains a lot of UVB. Thus, the evolution of skin color appears mainly to be a consequence of the body's need to preserve its vitamins.[422]

A common concern about vitamin D is the possibility of getting too much. If you get vitamin D from sunlight you won't have any problem getting too much vitamin D, although you should be concerned about sunburn and skin cancer. The reason is that the skin stops making vitamin D when the body's level gets high enough. The way to find out if you're getting enough vitamin D, either from sunlight or from supplements, is to get a blood test for vitamin D (25-hydroxyvitamin D, or 25-OH-D). This is a standard test that can be performed by any blood laboratory. A level below 30 nanograms per milliliter is thought to be inadequate, and a good level is in the range of

30–100 nanograms per milliliter. At this level, vitamin D helps to prevent many types of cancer. Some dermatologists recommend that people with light skin, who are at risk for skin damage from sunlight, should go out into the sunlight for twenty minutes to get their daily dose of vitamin D and then put on sunblock to prevent any further UVB exposure.[423] Thus, daily exposure to twenty minutes of sunlight is considered to do more good in preventing cancer than any potential harm of causing skin cancer.

A recent report by the Institute of Medicine (IOM) at the request of the United States government recommended that the daily recommended intake of vitamin D be raised to 600IU per day for most adults, with an upper recommended intake of 4,000IU.[424] The report based this level on bone health, but the recommendation excluded the known beneficial effects of vitamin D that promote health in body tissues and preventing diseases such as cancer and heart disease. Many nutritionists believe that although the increase in the recommended intake is in the right direction, it is not adequate for the health needs of most people. Vitamin D is not toxic for most people at 5,000–10,000IU per day, and there is an excellent body of knowledge about the proper intake levels necessary for the best health.[425] Therefore the IOM recommendation of 600IU per day is widely thought to be too low.[426]

For most people, an adequate dose of vitamin D is 25–50IU per pound per day, which for most adults is in the range of 2,000–10,000IU per day. To find out whether your dose is adequate, take about 2,000IU every day for several months during the winter, and then get a blood test. If it shows a level it the range of 40–60 nanograms per milliliter, that is enough. However if it's below 30, you should consider taking twice the dose, say, 4,000–5,000IU per day.[427] But don't make the mistake of assuming you're getting enough. Increasing your blood level of vitamin D by a factor of two, for example, from 20 nanograms per milliliter to 40, typically requires more than twice the original dose. Those who weigh 200 pounds or more may require 10,000IU per day or more to achieve a desirable blood level. Also, those who have a high fraction of body fat may need an even higher level, in the range 10,000 to 15,000IU.

Although you can get vitamin D from cod liver oil, this is not recommended as a source because cod liver oil contains enough vitamin A to cause vitamin A toxicity at a dosage level that would provide adequate vitamin D.[428] Milk is typically fortified with vitamin D at 100IU per cup, so to get enough vitamin D you would have to drink more than a gallon per day. Because vitamin D is fat-soluble, it is better absorbed when some fat is present in food eaten along with vitamin D tablets. Vitamin D supplements are readily available in 1,000, 2,000, and 5,000IU gelcaps. Considering their potential for better health, they are a remarkable bargain!

Calcium and Magnesium

Calcium and magnesium are necessary for healthy arteries, bones, muscles, and brain, as well as the retina. A deficiency in these important minerals can cause a variety of illnesses, such as osteomalacia or osteoporosis, and also high blood pressure and arterial inflammation. Calcium supplements are widely prescribed for older adults because without a good source of calcium in the diet such as dairy products or leafy green vegetables, many older people are deficient.[429] For the best effect, calcium should be taken in combination with magnesium and vitamin D. If you eat too much protein without enough carbohydrates, your body will metabolize the protein to synthesize blood sugar. This is likely to cause your body to excrete uric acid, which may take calcium along with it. If your diet doesn't contain enough calcium and magnesium, your body will take these important minerals from your bones.[430] This can induce a long-term deficit. For many individuals, such a deficit is an important contributor to osteomalacia and osteoporosis. When adequate magnesium is ingested it substitutes for calcium in the excretion of the metabolic products of protein, which prevents the loss of calcium and magnesium from the bones.

Magnesium is important for healthy arteries, muscles, bones, and the brain-in fact, it is essential for all organs including the eye.[431] A deficiency can cause high blood pressure, high cholesterol, irritability, fatigue, insomnia, muscle cramps, and eye twitching.[432] Magnesium helps balance the level of calcium in the blood indirectly by regulating the absorption of vitamin D, and directly by solubilizing calcium in the blood.[433] It is also a cellular signal essential in activating T-cells in the immune system.[434] Although a magnesium deficiency can cause a variety of symptoms such as neurologic and cardiac problems, it is difficult to diagnose. The symptoms of a magnesium deficiency are generally not specific to magnesium, and can also be caused by deficiencies of calcium, potassium, or other nutrients.[435]

Most of us are deficient in magnesium to some extent, because of widespread food processing in the modern world that removes the bran and germ of grains.[436] Stress in the modern lifestyle can cause the body to excrete more magnesium, leading to a deficiency that is hard to pinpoint. For those with diabetes, it is important to know that the disease causes the loss of more magnesium than in healthy people. Magnesium is required for the production and utilization of insulin, so the magnesium requirement for diabetics is higher. The body closely regulates the level of magnesium in the blood, even when the diet is deficient, so a deficiency usually doesn't show up on a blood test. To supply the blood and tissues with magnesium when there is a dietary deficiency, the body simply removes magnesium from the bones.[437] This is an important contributing factor for osteomalacia and osteoporosis, but it also has important consequences for the eye. The arteries of the eye are prone to damage from high blood pressure, a problem that can be readily alleviated with magnesium along with vitamin C and E. Once we are aware of the problem, it's easy to fix by getting more magnesium. An excellent diet and magnesium supplements can alleviate the deficiency and help prevent eye diseases associated with high blood pressure.

To recover from a calcium and/or magnesium deficit, you can take 500-1,000mg of calcium and 300–600mg of magnesium per day, depending on your body weight. Stated in terms of your body weight, the ideal amount of calcium is in the range of 4–8mg per pound per day, and the ideal amount of magnesium is 2.5–4.5mg per pound per day. The ideal ratio of the two is often quoted as two parts calcium to one part magnesium, for this is the ratio found in the bones, but a ratio of one to one is also commonly taken. You may need to take supplements for six to twelve months to allow your body to restore the levels in the tissues and bones.[438] Once your magnesium levels are raised, you can lower your supplement level by 50 percent to maintain them at a high level.

One recent concern is that excess calcium from supplements, especially in combination with vitamin D, may raise the calcium level too high, causing calcification of the arteries. You can prevent this problem by taking an adequate amount of magnesium with your calcium supplements. The magnesium tends to balance the blood level of calcium by helping to solubilize it, which helps the body restore it to the bones or excrete any excess.[439] Another concern when taking calcium and magnesium supplements is to make sure that the body can excrete any possible excess. Although a few hundred milligrams of these minerals may not seem very much, they otherwise can add up to an overdose if the doses you take over many weeks are greater than what your body needs.[440] Therefore, before you take calcium and magnesium supplements, consult your doctor to make sure your kidney function is adequate.

Good sources of calcium include dairy products, dark green leafy vegetables, fish with chewable bones such as salmon and sardines, rhubarb, and beans and legumes. For many people, a glass of milk at each meal provides an adequate amount of calcium, and for those who don't tolerate milk, yogurt is an excellent way to get calcium. However, most dairy products don't contain much magnesium.

Good sources of magnesium are seeds (for example, sunflower and pumpkin seeds), nuts, chocolate, leafy green vegetables, tomatoes, beans and legumes, and whole grains including wheat germ. Processed flour, even when enriched, contains very little magnesium, so try to avoid anything made from white of enriched flour, including white bread, cookies, crackers, cake, and most pastas, to maximize the magnesium you get from your diet. To get a perspective on the amount of magnesium in whole grain versus processed food, a slice of whole wheat bread can contain 25–50mg of magnesium. A cup of whole wheat flour contains 166mg of magnesium, but a cup of white enriched flour contains only 34Mg.[441] Because the body's requirement is on the order of 500mg per day, you can see the problem-we simply don't get enough in our modern diet. Whole-grain versions of most flour products are available, and if you are careful you can get enough magnesium by eating them. When you are tempted to eat processed food such as cake, for example, at a party, just remember to make up the deficit by eating more vegetables, or take a magnesium supplement the next day.

If you take calcium and magnesium supplements, remember that the type of calcium and magnesium is important. The reason is that some compounds, for example calcium carbonate, or magnesium oxide, although very widely used, are not well absorbed by most people. Only 30 percent of the calcium in calcium carbonate tablet, and 5–10 percent of the magnesium in a magnesium oxide tablet are typically absorbed.[442] One reason this form of magnesium is used so widely is that a tablet containing the same amount of magnesium is smaller compared to other forms, and many people find it easier to swallow. Preferable forms of calcium are lactate, malate, or chelate, and preferable forms of magnesium are lactate: malate, citrate, chelate, and chloride. These forms are better absorbed, and generally cost a little more, but the higher absorbability seems worth the extra expense. Magnesium chloride is absorbed best of the solid forms of magnesium. Magnesium oil, a supersaturated solution of magnesium chloride dissolved in water, can be applied to the skin and is readily absorbed.

Vitamin E

Vitamin E (tocopherols and tocotrienols) has been studied for many years, and is known to have several powerful effects.[443] One of them is its ability to prevent oxidation in cell membranes. It also regulates many other cellular mechanisms, for example, it inhibits aggregation and adhesion of blood platelets, which is beneficial for blood circulation.[444] Thus, it is not surprising that recently vitamin E was shown to decrease the risk of ischemic stroke, the type of stroke caused by blood clots. Also not surprising, and consistent with its effect of reducing blood clotting, are reports that vitamin E increases the risk of hemorrhagic stroke, in which blood leaks out of arteries.[445] When arteries are damaged by acute injury, inflammation, or low-grade scurvy (low vitamin C levels), they tend to break and bleed,[446] and the function of clotting is to stop bleeding. In other RCTs, vitamin E was found to increase all-cause mortality,[447] raising the question of what specifically might be its role. However, vitamin E was found to give a small increase in risk for strokes without any overall effect on mortality in another study,[448] pointing to its known role in slowing blood clotting. Patients taking "blood-thinning" drugs such as warfarin or aspirin to prevent blood clotting should consult a medical professional about the interaction between these drugs and vitamin E. When taking anticlotting drugs, it may be helpful to take vitamin E along with vitamin C, but also to reduce the dose of the anticlotting drugs for safety.

To put this information in perspective, ischemic stroke is four times more common than hemorrhagic stroke, so overall the effect of vitamin E is to reduce the risk for stroke.[449] Another perspective comes from an observational study showing that an adequate level of vitamin C in the bloodstream reduces the risk of stroke by more than 50 percent, and even more for those who are hypertensive or overweight.[450] More recently, another perspective on vitamin E and stroke was provided by an RCT showing that six month treatment with vitamin C, vitamin E, coenzyme Q_{10}, and selenium increased elasticity of both the large and small arteries, improved glucose and fat metabolism, and reduced blood pressure.[451] Therefore, taking vitamin E along with vitamin C and other helpful antioxidants and nutrients can greatly reduce the risk of stroke, lower blood pressure, and improve overall health.

The specific biochemical functions of vitamin E in the body are not yet known.[452] Vitamin E has been described as the only antioxidant that is also an important cell-signaling molecule.[453] Vitamin E is known to inhibit protein-kinase C, is a cell-signaling molecule that is involved in inhibiting growth of smooth muscle cells, and thus an important signal in the growth of cancer. Although its beneficial effects have long been known, vitamin E is not just one biochemical. The d-alpha-tocopherol form is thought to be selectively taken up by the body, so it is the most widely available. However, vitamin E exists in eight different forms, including alpha-, beta-, delta-and gamma-tocopherols and tocotrienols.[454] The different forms of vitamin E are all antioxidants, but are thought to have unique functions in the body.[455] For example, they can prevent oxidative stress, reduce cardiovascular inflammation, and reduce cancel rates.[456] For acute symptoms, a topical application of tocopherols and tocotrienols to the eye can provide a higher level in the ocular tissues than oral administration.[457] Tocotrienols function to inhibit cholesterol synthesis, assimilate better into brain tissue, and are more potent antioxidants than tocopherols.[458] Although they are more expensive than tocopherols, their benefit may be worth the expense. It seems likely that simply taking a supplement of d-alpha-tocopherol is missing a large part of the benefit-it is probably more helpful to take a mixture of tocopherols and tocotrienols.

Another problem that has confounded the interpretation of studies administering vitamin E has been the use of synthetic dl-alpha-tocopherol,[459] which, although it is an antioxidant of the same power, hat only half of the biological activity of the natural form d-alpha-tocopherol.[460] The interpretation of the beneficial effects of vitamin E has been also complicated by differing results in studies of vitamin E that have given different doses for different durations. These may not have taken into account other confounding factors such as existing vitamin E levels and related diseases.[461] For example, in some RCTs testing the effect of vitamin E on age-related eye disease, the participants took multivitamin tablets that contain vitamin E.[462] But this was not fully taken into account in the initial reports, tending to confound the conclusions of the study.

A further problem with the interpretation of many studies is that a low dose of vitamin E, taken in isolation over the short term, will likely not show its full benefit because, as explained above, vitamin E is known to be synergistic with vitamin C and other antioxidants such as selenium. For example, vitamin C circulating in the bloodstream can regenerate vitamin E from its inactive oxidized form into its active reduced form, greatly extending the effect of the vitamin E dose.[463] While some benefits of vitamin E, such as its effect on reducing cardiovascular inflammation, are evident within a few months, much of the benefit in preventing age-related eye disease is thought to become most apparent over decades. A combination of essential nutrients such as vitamin C, vitamin E, zinc, and selenium, along with other nutrients such as coenzyme Q_{10}, alpha-lipoic acid, and glutathione will likely provide a synergistic effect, that is, the result will be greater than all the nutrients taken separately. The results from an RCT depend to a great extent on how the scientific question is stated. When a study attempts to discover the role of a single nutrient, ostensibly to simplify the question, the result may not be very helpful in understanding its role in the diet in the presence of additional nutrients. When placed in perspective, the overall evidence about the effect of supplemental vitamin E seems clear-it helps improve cardiovascular and eye heath as part of a balanced diet and regime of supplements.

Vitamin E has long been considered a safe vitamin when it is taken over many years at doses widely used to prevent disease (400–3,200IU per day).[464] It prolongs the life of mice by reducing cancer rates when it is taken long-term.[465] It is actively metabolized at high levels and does not accumulate in the liver,[466] so it is safe to take over long periods. You may be advised to avoid taking vitamin E if you have a late stage of retinitis pigmentosa (see Chapter 5), but together with vitamin C, the overall evidence shows that vitamin E is helpful in preventing many eye diseases and for cardiovascular health. An obvious preventive measure for the anticlotting effect of vitamin E in promoting hemorrhagic strokes is to build up the dose slowly (over several months). This allows it to strengthen the cardiovascular system as a part of a healthy diet, which should include vitamin

C in sufficient doses (3,000-10,000mg per day in divided doses). This combination of vitamins C and E will strengthen collagen throughout the body, increase artery elasticity, lower blood pressure, and prevent strokes and cardiovascular inflammation.[467] Those with cardiovascular problems or taking anticoagulants should consult with their doctor before taking large doses of vitamin E.

Vitamin K

Another vitamin important to the eye is vitamin K. It is essential for blood clotting and regulation of calcium in remodeling bone and in calcium excretion. Vitamin K is a fat-soluble cofactor for several reactions in which proteins newly synthesized by cells are modified for their roles in building and maintenance of the body. These proteins are important for coagulation of blood platelets, for bone and cartilage construction and metabolism, and for several other essential functions.[468] Vitamin K is thought to be important for maintaining the elasticity of the trabecular meshwork that regulates eye pres-sure.[469] The trabecular meshwork is a spongy filter that resists the flow of aqueous humor out of the eye. When it doesn't function properly or when it gets clogged with debris, ocular pressure can rise. This is a primary cause for glaucoma. Therefore maintenance of the trabecular meshwork by vitamin K is crucial to preserve its softness and elasticity. The meshwork is thought to respond dynamically to specific conditions with expression of different combinations of genes. Some of the gene expression requires vitamin K.[470] Also, vitamin K helps to maintain the aging inner retina, near the ganglion cells.[471] Vitamin K is made by bacteria in the gut, but a large proportion comes from the diet. It is found in leafy green vegetables (collards, kale, spinach, Brussels sprouts, broccoli, cabbage, and turnip, beet, mustard, and dandelion greens), onions, kiwi fruit, and citrus. The dietary reference intake (DRI) for vitamin K is 100 micrograms (mcg), which is obtained from one serving of greens or broccoli. If a large quantity is eaten it can be stored in the body for future use. Eating food containing a large amount of vitamin K is safe, but talk to your doctor before taking it if you have any special medical conditions.

Iron

Another important factor in age-related eye disease is the amount of iron in the bloodstream and in eye tissues. Iron is a very important nutrient, and it is crucial for every cell in the body. Most of the body's iron is within molecules such as hemoglobin in red blood cells and myoglobin in muscles.[472] The function of these molecules is to carry oxygen from the bloodstream into the tissues, such as the muscles; that need it to help generate energy from blood sugar. Other molecules that contain iron are the enzymes, such as cytochromes, responsible for metabolic reactions in every cell.

When the body has an iron deficiency it is unable to generate enough red blood cells to carry oxygen to its tissues, and the tissues become less efficient at generating energy necessary for growth and maintenance. Iron deficiencies are important, and they are common when blood is lost or when the dies is deficient. It is fairly easy to correct an iron deficiency, because red meat, liver, and turkey contain generous amounts. This form of iron, called "heme-bound iron," is readily absorbed by the gut.

It is easy to get too much iron, however, because the body has no known way to excrete it.[473] Excess iron in the bloodstream is absorbed by the liver and other tissues and stored in granules of ferritin, a special iron-binding protein. This provides some iron-buffering capacity to lessen the effect of an excess or a deficiency of iron in the diet. For this and other unknown reasons, iron naturally tends to build of in cells with age.[474] In some individuals, iron builds up to toxic levels in the tissues, a condition called iron overload or hemochromatosis. The cure is to reduce iron intake by eating less red meat, or in severe cases, by blood-letting at regular intervals.

Unbound iron is known to produce oxidative stress similar to that caused by oxygen and light. As described earlier, the iron-containing cytochromes inside retinal can generate oxidative stress when they absorb light. The lipofuscin granules in RPE cells are thought to be caused in part by oxidation from unbound or "labile" iron.[475] The buildup of lipofuscin happens in cells that are not actively dividing, such as retinal neurons. Overall, this means that iron builds up in retinal cells with age, causing damage that increases with age, which causes a buildup of lipofuscin granules and damage to the RPE cell; whose job it is to deal with cellular garbage.[476]

Paradoxically, oxidative stress has been linked to too little iron as well as too much. When rats were given a large dose of iron, equivalent to what is recommended for pregnant women, they had an elevated level of ethane, a product of lipid peroxidation, a form of oxidative stress.[477] But rats already deficient it iron that were not given additional iron in supplements, also showed a similar increase in oxidative stress. This suggests that it is very important to get an adequate amount of iron, but not too much or too little.

The body has no known mechanism for actively excreting excess iron, and typically an adult man passively excretes only 1mg of iron per day.[478] Heme-bound iron is readily absorbed through a special transport pathway, but this absorption is not closely regulated. This means that when you eat red meat, you absorb virtually all of the iron in the meat, so eating too much red meat can be a risk for many age-related diseases. Other forms of iron, such as that found in spinach, chocolate, beans, lentils, and tomato products are called "nonheme iron" because they are not bound to hemoglobin and myoglobin found in meat. However, because the proper level of iron is so important for the body, the absorption of nonheme bound iron is closely regulated.[479] The gut regulates the amount of iron absorbed by preferentially absorbing nonheme iron when the body has an iron deficiency.[480] Iron is carried in the blood by a special protein, transferrin, that binds it tightly. This keeps the free iron content of the blood low. Once in the bloodstream, iron from both heme and non-heme origin competes for absorption into new red blood cells.

A standard component of routine blood tests is the "hematocrit;" a measurement of the red blood cell content of your blood and a good indicator of the amount of iron in your body. The iron supplement dose you require depends on how much iron you absorb from food.[481] Iron is an important nutrient, but when we get too much, the body ages more quickly, and this often shows up first in the eye. If you have a high level of iron in your blood, you can reduce it by eating less red meat and avoiding multivitamin tablets that contain iron. This will keep you healthier, reduce oxidative stress, and prevent premature aging. If your diet is deficient in iron, a dose of up to 10mg per day is recommended for men and up to 20mg per day is recommended for women of childbearing age.

Zinc, Copper, and Selenium

After iron, zinc is the most abundant trace element in the body. It is essential as a catalyst for dozens of enzyme reactions, in protein folding, in regulation of gene expression, and it is thought to have protective role in cardiovascular disease.[482] For all of these reasons, zinc is important for the eye. It is found at relatively high concentrations in the retina, especially in the pigment epithelium, and it is necessary cofactor in the metabolism of retinal, the visual pigment.[483] In observational studies, a high level of zinc intake reduced the risk for macular degeneration. Older people are often zinc-deficient likely because of deficiencies in their diet and absorption. A zinc deficiency is difficult to diagnose because the blood level is not a good indication of the body's stores. The body stores enough zinc for several months, so a quick increase or decrease in intake will not affect the body's stores or the blood level much. However, zinc deficiency is common among individuals older than sixty-five years of age.[484]

Zinc is found in many vegetables, meats, and whole grains, but it is typically missing in processes foods because, like magnesium, it is contained mostly in the germ and bran. A zinc supplement of 20 ml per day is commonly taken, and up to 80mg per day has been taken to help prevent macular degeneration.[485] When taken at this higher dosage, zinc should be taken with copper at 2mg per day to prevent copper depletion by the higher level of zinc.[486]

Copper is necessary for a variety of biochemical reactions in the body. Copper is toxic when more that a few milligrams per day is taken, and a well-balanced diet based on vegetables and fruits ordinarily provides enough, so additional copper supplements should be avoided. Red meat contains a plentiful amount, so as with iron, eating a lot of meat can cause a copper overdose. If zinc and copper supplements are taken they should also be combined with beta-carotene, vitamin C, and vitamin E for the greatest reduction in risk for disease.

Selenium is another trace element known to be helpful in boosting the immune system[487] and preventing eye disease. Just a little selenium can greatly increase the effectiveness of vitamin E,[488] which can help to lower oxidative stress in the photoreceptors. Good sources of selenium are fish, liver, meat, eggs, whole wheat, beans, and nuts. Plants do not need selenium so the level of selenium they contain depends on the soil in which they grow.[489] Soils in the MIdwest contain an adequate amount of selenium, but soils in the Eastern and Northwestern states are deficient, so grains and livestock raised there tend to have inadequate levels of selenium.[490]

A typical selenium supplement is 50 to 200 micrograms (mcg) per day. However, it is easy to get a toxic overdose if a vitamin and mineral supplement contains a high dose of selenium (greater than 200mcg).[491] Watch out for Brazil nuts, which contain as much as 540mcg per ounce (six to eight nuts).[492] When taking a multivitamin supplement along with Brazil nuts, it's easy to get too much selenium. Typical overdose symptoms are brittle nails or hair. Depending on the amount of overdose, the level of selenium takes several weeks to months to build up in the body, and nails take several weeks to months to grow out. Therefore, if you are getting too much selenium it may take several months to notice. If you're taking a multivitamin supplement that contains more than 50mcg of selenium, limit your intake of Brazil nuts to one per day, or even one every other day.

Selenium at levels below 400mcg per day is known to be helpful in preventing disease such as prostate cancer[493] and infections such as colds or flu. To reduce your risk of macular degeneration, you can take supplements of selenium (50-200mcg per day), in combination with zinc, copper, beta-carotene, vitamin C, and vitamin E.[494]

Ultra-Trace Minerals

Several minerals are thought to be essential in the diet at extremely low levels. These minerals include arsenic, boron, fluoride, manganese, molybdenum, nickel, silicon, and vanadium.[495] They are utilized as cofactors of enzymes and can generally be acquired in a well-balanced diet. At high levels, they can be toxic, but the body needs a small quantity for health. Because many of them are essential for the brain they are necessary for optimal eye health as well. A good way to get ultratrace minerals is to use sea salt, which contains a mixture of a wide variety of elements.

Omega-3 and Omega-6 Fatty Acids

Although we have heard much about avoiding fat in our diet, several polyunsaturated fatty acids an necessary for growth and maintenance of tissues throughout the body. Omega-3 and omega-6 fatty acid; are required by all cells for their membranes and biochemical reactions. In our modern diet, a deficit o omega-3 fatty acids is very common because most seed oils like canola, olive, corn, or peanut oils are high in omega-6 but low in omega-3 fatty acids. A deficit in omega-3 fatty acids is a risk factor for heart disease, eye diseases, and other diseases of biochemical origin like pellagra. This is currently an important topic for research.

Omega-3 fatty acids include alpha-linolenic acid (ALA or LNA), eicosapentaenoic acid (EPA), and docosahexaenoic acid (DHA). All three of these fatty acids are necessary for cells, but the body can make EPA and DHA from ALA, so of the three only ALA is essential. However, the conversion from. ALA/LNA to EPA and DHA is slow, so all three of these oils are helpful to prevent a deficiency. A point of confusion to note is that another biochemical, alpha-lipoic acid (a different but useful fatty acid and, powerful antioxidant), has the same appreviation, ALA, so it is often confused with alpha-linolenic acid Also, alpha-linolenic acid, which is an essential omega-3 fatty acid, is different than alpha-linoleic acid, an essential omega-6 oil.

Omega-3 oils are especially important for photoreceptors in the eye, because the photoreceptor outer segments, which are continually being regrown, contain the highest fraction of DHA in any cell of the body. Thirty to fifty percent of fatty acid molecules in the outer segments are DHA.[496] These polyunsaturated fatty acids are prone to oxidation by oxygen, light, and environmental toxins, which is thought to be an initiating step in many age-related eye diseases such as macular degeneration and retinitis pigmentosa. A diet high in omega-3 fatty acids increases the amount of DHA found in the outer segments, which appears to be helpful in preserving photoreceptor function.[497]

The ratio of omega-3 to omega-6 fatty acids in the diet is important because it determines how available each type is for cell growth and maintenance. Historically the ratio was nearly even, but in our modern diet the fraction of omega-6 fatty acids is greater, typically by a factor of fifteen to twenty. This is thought to contribute to heart disease and complications of diabetes. Although omega-6 fatty acids arc necessary in our diet, most of us need more omega-3 fatty acids to keep the balance right. An excellent source of omega-3 fatty acids is oily fish (EPA and DHA: salmon, trout, tuna, anchovies, sardines, and mackerel), and range-fed beef, lamb, and chicken.[498] Remember that the smaller fish, like anchovies and sardines, have the lowest content of toxins and heavy metals such as mercury because they are lower or the food chain. A four-ounce serving of oily fish provides a good way to get omega-3 oils (salmon 1,000–1,500mg; sardines and mackerel, 2,000–3,300mg), and many fish oil supplements are available in softgel capsules.

The essential omega-3 oil, ALA, can be obtained from some vegetable sources such as flaxseed oil, walnuts, lecithin, and wheat germ. Flaxseed oil is most commonly taken because its content of ALA is, relatively high. Many doctors also advise that to help prevent heart disease, taking a handful of walnut: at each meal is useful as a source of ALA. Note that flaxseed oil, also known as linseed oil, is highly reactive with oxygen because it is a polyunsaturated oil, and spoils quickly. It can cause a fire from the heat of oxidation if it is left to dry in an oil-soaked tightly crumpled rag or paper towel. Also, note that commercial "boiled linseed oil" is inedible because it contains metal additives. Flaxseed oil should be kept in a black bottle in the refrigerator, because it can go rancid in as little as two or three months if it is stored at room temperature in a bottle that has been opened and exposed to air and/or light. This is, of course, what also happens to these fatty acids when they are in your photoreceptors: they are readily oxidized by toxic chemicals, oxygen, and light. When flaxseed oil is fresh it smells nutty, and you can tell when it goes rancid because it smells bad. Flaxseed oil sold in softgel capsules is more stable and can stage fresh on your cabinet shelf for as long as six months.

Remember that flaxseed oil readily oxidizes when heated, so it should not be used for cooking. You can prevent a bottle of flaxseed oil from going rancid so quickly by adding the contents of a few 400IU capsules of d-alpha-tocopherol (the nonacetate form of vitamin E).[499] You can make your own flaxseed oil by grinding flaxseeds into a fine paste using manual or electric flaxseed mill, coffee grinder, or blender. If the seeds are fresh, the oil from the seed is, less rancid than flaxseed oil you store for weeks in a bottle. The grinding operation is necessary in order for the oil to be absorbed by the gut.

Lutein, Zeaxanthin, and Other Carotenoids

These important carotenoid pigments are antioxidants found in the eye. Zeaxanthin is a stereoisomer o lutein, that is, they have the same chemical structure, but their shapes are mirror images (identical but reversed). They are thought to lessen oxidative stress in the central part of the retina. They appear to have two roles: The first is to form the macular pigment, which is a yellow-orange filter that removes blue light that would otherwise fall on the center of the retina. In this role, they are oxidized by blue light, and so must be replaced continually. The second role is as an antioxidant that can quench oxygen radicals continuously, without a requirement to be regenerated by another antioxidant.

The body cannot make lutein or zeaxanthin, so they are essential biochemicals that must be obtained in the diet.[500] A deficiency of lutein and/or zeaxanthin early in life causes structural problems in the RPE cells, which may contribute to macular degeneration. However, lutein and zeaxanthin are thought to reverse (to some extent) damage caused by their deficiency if they are taken later in life, when the deposits of lipofuscin that cause macular degeneration appear.[501] They are also anti-inflammatory, which is important for the eye because many eye diseases are started by inflammation.[502]

Lutein and zeaxanthin are the principal yellow-orange pigments in corn, peppers, and green leafy vegetables such as collards, kale, and spinach. Although these vegetables are also good sources of vitamin A, the body cannot convert between these nutrients and vitamin A, so a dietary source of both is, essential. A diet supplemented with lutein and zeaxanthin lowers the risk for eye disease.[503] An effective dose of lutein for reducing risk for eye disease is 12mg per day, which is roughly the amount in one-hall cup of spinach or collards.[504] Because macular degeneration starts early in life and accelerates with age, it is particularly important to have a diet rich in lutein and zeaxanthin during your entire adult life. One concern is that if high levels of lutein are ingested, the skin turns yellowish from the carotenoid pigment. This is harmless and reversible, for if you reduce your intake the skin will return to its normal color.[505] Although the benefits of supplementation with lutein and zeaxanthin are clear in the laboratory and it clinical studies, large RCTs have not found a benefit yet. However, many eye doctors are recommending them because there appears to be little risk from these important carotenoids.[506]

Another carotenoid is astaxanthin, a reddish carotenoid found in salmon, shrimp, and yeast, that is a powerful antioxidant.[507] It is helpful for preventing oxidative stress, and is thought to help prevent inflammation in blood vessels. Along with other carotenoids and an excellent diet, this may help prevent retinal damage in glaucoma and diabetic retinopathy.

Lipoic Acid

Another powerful antioxidant that is thought to help prevent eye disease is lipoic acid.[508] Although it is not an essential nutrient, it is an important cofactor for enzymes in metabolic pathways, including in the retina. In a laboratory study, rats given lipoic acid had less damage from oxidative stress, especially from injury to blood vessels such as the damage caused in glaucoma to retinal blood vessels.[509] Lipoic acid ha, been used to treat neuropathic pain in diabetics.[510] It is transported into epithelial cells such as those or the surface of the cornea, along with vitamin B_5 and biotin,[511] implying that these nutrients are required together.

Lipoic acid is a master antioxidant, similar to other antioxidants such as glutathione that are useed widely throughout the body. Because lipoic acid is well absorbed from supplements, it is an excellent way to reduce oxidative stress.[512] Lipoic acid prevents the depletion of other antioxidants by reducing oxidative stress throughout the tissues of the body, and it is thought to be synergistic with other antioxidants such as vitamin C, vitamin E, zinc and selenium.[513] For these reasons supplementation with lipoic acid is an excellent way to extend the usefulness of other antioxidants such as vitamin C an(vitamin E. It can regenerate vitamin C, or alternately can prevent vitamin C or vitamin E from being oxidized.[514] Lipoic acid is therefore thought to be useful in preventing glaucoma and cataract.[515] Typical doses are 100 to 200mg, several times daily, but larger doses up to several thousand mg per day are helpful and reasonable when indicated by symptoms of stress.[516] A recent study showed that topical application of alpha-lipoic acid raised its concentration in the eye, suggesting that this may be effective in treating eye disease.[517]

Coenzyme Q_{10}

Coenzyme Q_{10} (CoQ_{10}) is a fat-soluble cofactor important for the metabolism of every cell in the body, and is also an antioxidant.[518] Like many B vitamins, it is necessary for the production of adenosine triphosphate (ATP), the primary molecule that supplies energy to run cells. CoQ_{10} is more effective at preventing oxidation of lipids than vitamin E or the carotenoids.[519] It can act in synergy with other antioxidants, because it can help to regulate and regenerate vitamin E. CoQ_{10} is not a vitamin because cells can normally synthesize enough of it. However, the level of CoQ_{10} drops in the aging eye, and this loss of CoQ_{10}, along with its antioxidant and metabolic properties, is thought to be linked to a higher risk for macular degeneration. Good sources of CoQ_{10} are meat, fish, nuts, and some oils, and it is present at low levels in fruits and vegetables, dairy products, and whole-grains. CoQ_{10} supplements (100–1,000mg per day) are used widelyand are safe at high doses.[520]

N-Acetylcysteine, Glutathione

Glutathione is a powerful antioxidant synthesized in the body and used widely by the body to protect against oxidative stress. The level of glutathione in the blood and tissues is commonly taken to indicate the antioxidant state of the body.[521] However, glutathione is not effective when taken orally because it is not well absorbed. N-acetyl-cysteine, a precursor for glutathione, is commonly taken to increase glutathione levels in the body. N-acetylcysteine is helpful for the oil glands that surround the eye and limit the spread of tears,[522] and it helps prevent inflammation when it is applied topically after laser keratectomy.[523] It is also helpful in protecting the RPE cells,[524] and in preventing retinal detachment.[525] Although N-acetylcysteine is thought to be safe for most people in doses up to 1,000mg per day, you should consult a medical professional before taking it. Normally it is taken along with vitamin C and other antioxidants.

A recent development is that liposomal glutathione supplements have become available to supplement the body's intrinsic ability to synthesize this important antioxidant. This form of glutathione is encapsulated within liposomes, nanosized spheres of lipid molecules called phospholipids. Glutathione is necessary in all cells and especially helpful in supporting brain function. Liposomal glutathione is absorbed at a much higher rate than plain glutathione, and enter the bloodstream directly to support this body's internal glutathione levels. This form of glutathione, though more expensive, is thought to be superior to the standard form for the prevention and recovery from many eye diseases.

COMMON BENEFITS OF SUPPLEMENTS

Given our current knowledge about the risk of eye disease due to nutritional deficiencies and from oxidative stress, the best advice appears to be to eat an excellent diet and take supplements for nutrient that have been shown to be effective in a multitude of studies over the past seventy years. However, the necessary randomized controlled trials to test the optimal combinations and levels of supplements have not been performed for many essential nutrients. This raises the question about the proper rationale for eye disease prevention and treatment. Should one simply heed the standard conservative advice to wait until more is known before taking supplements?[526] The evidence presented in this book strongly suggests that one should not wait. It is important to start eating an excellent diet and, where necessary, taking nutritional supplements early in life because deficiencies in nutrients over many decades are directly linked to eye disease. This will prevent problems with oxidative stress on the tissues of the eye, so they don't build up to the point of disease. Many observational studies have shown beneficial effects of vitamin C and vitamin E, especially when they are taken together with other antioxidants such as beta-carotene, lutein and zeaxanthin, alpha-lipoic acid, zinc, and selenium. The main points can already be understood and followed: eat a healthy diet and take supplements at an adequate dose, and you will see the benefit over your lifetime.

It is apparent from the evidence that many eye diseases have a common root-age-related oxidative stress-that originates from several causes. This suggests treatment with a common set of antioxidant supplements that are good for preventing a variety of specific conditions.[527] The aging eye has lower levels of antioxidants such as coenzyme Q_{10} (CoQ_{10}) and vitamin C, and this is thought to be a factor in age-related eye disease.[528] Antioxidants such as vitamin C, vitamin E, selenium, CoQ_{10}, glutathione, and alpha-lipoic acid act in symbiosis, where a low level of one of these can be made up by sufficient levels of the others.[529] Glutathione can help to recycle vitamin C from its oxidized form to its active reduced form,[530] and vitamin C can help to recycle both glutathione and vitamin E.[531]

One might imagine that an advanced degree is necessary to understand the intricacies of how nutrients affect the body and eye to get a benefit from nutrient supplements. However, finding what combinations and doses of supplements are optimal does not need to be too difficult or complex, Knowledge about the effects of nutrition on age-related oxidative stress in eye disease is quickly gaining momentum,[532] and we will learn more about which combination of nutrients is best for each eye condition as more trials of dietary and supplemental nutrients are published. However, picking the proper combination of nutrients seems clear even now, because the efficacy and safety of vitamins and nutrients-when taken in the proper doses-is well known. If you have a special condition or need, you should consult a nutrition-aware medical professional for precautions and to determine doses. Most people can benefit greatly by taking generous doses of vitamins and nutrients. The orthomolecular literature offers helpful guidance.[533] Antioxidants are known to be synergistic, and it seems likely that combination that maximally protects against cataract, for example, may also be effective in protecting against retinitis pigmentosa and macular degeneration.

ORTHOMOLECULAR DOSES OF NUTRIENTS TO PREVENT EYE DISEASE

Orthomolecular medicine emphasizes the need to take adequate doses of nutrients.[534] They should be taken according to the nutritional needs of the individual, which may vary widely. This can be done in program of preventative medicine along with a "nutrition-aware" medical professional. Although the DRI for nutrients prevents the symptoms of acute deficiency, additional amounts of nutrients allow the body's metabolic reactions to proceed more fully, providing a greater health benefit.[535] Each individual; need for nutrients such as vitamins C and E differs, depending on his or her unique genetics biochemistry, diet, and level of stress and disease.[536] Vitamin C (ascorbate) cannot be synthesized by humans, primates, and guinea pigs, but most other animal species make 10–20gm each day (relative to human body weight), and they make more when they are stressed physically or by disease.[537] Typically vitamin C is taken up to bowel tolerance, which for a healthy individual is an oral dose of 2,000–10,000mg per day. However, when disease or oxidative stress affects the body, the gut absorbs more ascorbate according to the body's need, typically up to approximately tenfold more.[538] Vitamin E has been shown to be safe and effective for most people at high doses (800–3,200IU per day) to prevent oxidative stress and disease.[539] The benefit in reducing oxidative stress is likely to be more obvious with these "mega" doses. A collection of nutrients, including antioxidants, when taken in combination and dosed according to the individual's need will likely multiply the beneficial effects. A typical daily supplement plan to help an adult prevent many eye diseases would include:

Vitamin A	5,000–10,000IU
Beta-carotene	10–20 milligrams (mg)
Thiamine (B_1)	50–100mg
Riboflavin (B_2)	50–100mg
Niacin (B_3)	50–2,000mg, divided doses
Pantothenate (B_5)	50–100mg
Pyridoxine (B_6)	50–100mg
Biotin (B_7)	50–100 micrograms (mcg)
Folate (B_9)	400–2,000mcg
Cobalamin (B_{12})	100–1,000mcg when necessary

Vitamin C	3,000–10,000mg (15–50mg/pound/day), divided doses, to bowel tolerance
Vitamin D	2,000–10,000IU (20–50IU/pound/day)
Vitamin E	400–1,200IU mixed tocopherols, tocotrienols
Calcium	500–1,000mg (2–5mg/pound/day), as chelate, lactate, malate
Magnesium	300–600mg (1.5–3mg/pound/day), as chloride, chelate, or malate
Iron	2–20mg, depending on need
Zinc	20–50mg
Copper	2mg
Selenium	50–200mcg
Lutein/Zeaxanthin	10–20mg (1/2 cup kale, collards, or spinach)
Omega-3 oils	1,000–3,000mg (1–2 teaspoons flaxseed oil, fish oil)
Alpha-lipoic acid	200–1,000mg
Coenzyme Q_{10}	100–1,000mg
N-acetylcysteine	100–500mg, check for contraindi-cations
Trace elements	Sea salt

A good way to organize this supplement plan is to take a multivitamin-mineral tablet that contains most of the nutrients listed, and then take additional tablets or foods for vitamin C, D,

E, calcium, magnesium, lutein, zeaxanthin, omega-3 oils, alpha-lipioic acid, and N-acetylcysteine.

SUMMARY: A COMBINATION OF NUTRIENTS IS MOST EFFECTIVE

We know that supplemental antioxidants and nutrients are effective in preventing eye disease from literally thousands of studies over the past half-century. Usually they are more effective when they are taken in combination than when one or two are taken alone. Thus, vitamins A, B_1, B_2, B_3, B_5, B_6, B_7, B_9, B_{12}, C, and E, carotenoids (lutein and zeaxanthin), zinc, selenium, calcium, magnesium, lipoic acid, and omega-3 fatty acids can do much to prevent or delay the onset of typical age-related eye diseases when they are taken at the proper levels and in combination with a diet containing lots of fruits, whole grains, and leafy green vegetables over a decade or more.[540] Zinc is found in relatively high concentrations in the retina and is necessary for several enzyme systems to preserve health. Selenium in the proper amount i; an important antioxidant and can help to prevent macular degeneration. Supplemental calcium and magnesium can correct very common deficiencies and help to reduce blood pressure, maintain health of arteries, and prevent retinopathy. The carotenoids are helpful in preventing light from reaching the macular photoreceptors, and are antioxidants that help to prevent oxidation caused by light. Vitamin E is helpful in reducing oxidation of fatty acids in cell membranes, which is very important for reducing damage to the retina and its photoreceptors. Vitamin C is helpful in strengthening capillary blood vessels and to neutralize free radicals, and it helps the body to regenerate vitamin E. Vitamin C is also helpful in reducing oxidation of all the tissues of the eye, and in reducing ocular pressure to prevent glaucoma, Although proper nutrition is not a panacea, when you eat an excellent diet along with selected supplements of vitamins and nutrients (consulting with your medical professional if you have special needs), these nutrients can do much to prevent diseases of the eye and in the rest of the body. They are most effective when taken at a sufficient level starting early in life.

Progress in the science of nutrition is certain to discover more of the details about the essential nutrients and the best combinations of them to prevent disease. Studies to test the benefits of nutrition and supplements have often been difficult to interpret when one or several nutrients are tested at a low dose. However, it seems inevitable that as better knowledge about nutrition is accumulated, the advantage of taking adequate doses of nutrients will be better understood by the administrators of health studies. Studies will begin testing different combinations to find the best for each condition as the advantage of taking the proper combinations of nutrients becomes more widely understood. New health studies will provide knowledge about the best combinations of nutrients for each organ in the body including the eye.

Although the references in this book are current, it seems likely that new reports will supersede those we rely on today as the literature of nutrition progresses. This will not obviate our current knowledge but will extend it. As access to health science improves, for example, with freely available articles on the Internet, new reports about the benefits of nutrition are sure to enhance our health further. Medical professionals are rapidly learning to assimilate this new knowledge, including the basic concepts o orthomolecular medicine. This is part of a healthy lifestyle we can follow. So, as Andrew Saul explained in 2003, we are in control of what we eat, which allows us to take charge of our health. Nowhere is the more obvious than in treating eye disease with vitamins.

REFERENCES

Chapter 1. How Vitamins Can Help Our Health: An Introduction

[1] Saul, A. *Doctor Yourself. Natural Healing That Works.* Laguna Beach, CA: Basic Health Publications, 2003.

[2] Fine, L.C., J.S. Heier. *The Aging Eye: Preventing and Treating Eye Disease.* Special Health Reports. Boston, MA: Harvard Medical School, 2010.

[3] Ames, B.N. "Optimal Micronutrients Delay Mitochondrial Decay and Age-associated Diseases." *Mech Ageing Dev* 131 (2010):473–479.

[4] Esselstyn, C.B. *Prevent and Reverse Heart Disease: The Revolutionary, Scientifically Proven, Nutrition-Based Cure.* New York, NY: Avery, 2008. Campbell, T.C., T.M. Campbell, II. *The China Study: The Most Comprehensive Study of Nutrition Ever Conducted and Startling Implications for Diet, Weight Loss, and Long-Term Health.* Dallas, TX: Ben-Bella Books, 2006.

[5] Pollan, M. *In Defense of Food: An Eater's Manifesto.* New York, NY: Penguin, 2009.

[6] Ames, B.N. "Low Micronutrient Intake May Accelerate the Degenerative Diseases of Aging through Allocation of Scarce Micronutrients by

Triage." *Proc Natl Acad Sci USA.* 103 (2006):17589–17594.

[7] Harper, A.E. "Defining the Essentiality of Nutrients." Chapter 1 in *Modern Nutrition in Health and Disease,* editors M.E. Shils, J.A. Olson, M. Shike, et al., 9th ed. Baltimore, MD: Williams & Wilkins, 1999.

[8] Pauling, L. "Orthomolecular Psychiatry. Varying the Concentrations of Substances Normally Present in the Human Body May Control Mental Disease." *Science* 160(825) (Apr 19, 1968):265–271. Pauling, L. *How to Live Longer And Feel Better.* Corvallis, OR: Oregon State University Press, 1986, 2006.

[9] Hoffer, A., A.W. Saul. *Orthomolecular Medicine for Everyone: Megavitamin Therapeutics for Families and Physicians.* Laguna Beach, CA: Basic Health Publications, 2008. Hickey, S., A.W. Saul. *Vitamin C: The Real Story, the Remarkable and Controversial Healing Factor.* Laguna Beach, CA: Basic Health Publications, 2008.

[10] Ames, B.N. "Low Micronutrient Intake May Accelerate the Degenerative Diseases of Aging through Allocation of Scarce Micronutrients by Triage." *Proc Natl Acad Sci USA.* 103 (2006):17589–17594.

[11] Pauling, L. *How to Live Longer And Feel Better.* Corvallis, OR: Oregon State University Press, 1986, 2006.

[12] Hoffer, A., A.W. Saul. *Orthomolecular Medicine for Everyone: Megavitamin Therapeutics for Families and Physicians.* Laguna Beach, CA: Basic Health Publications, 2008.

[13] Dean, C. *The Magnesium Miracle.* New York, NY: Ballantine, 2007.

[14] Phillips, J.B., R. Muheim, P.E. Jorge. "A Behavioral Perspective on the Biophysics of the Light-Dependent Magnetic Compass: a Link between Directional and Spatial Perception?" *J Exp Biol* 213 (Oct 1, 2010):3247–3255.

[15] Orbach, D.N., B. Fenton. "Vision Impairs the Abilities of Bats to Avoid Colliding with Stationary Obstacles." *PLoS One* 5 (11) (2010):e13912.

[16] Davis, A. *Let's Eat Right to Keep Fit.* Rev. ed. New York, NY: Harcourt, Brace, Jovanovich, 1970.

[17] Carson, R. *Silent Spring.* 1st Mariner Books ed. Boston, MA: Houghton Mifflin, 2002.

[18] Saleh, S., R.N. Haddadin, S. Baillie, et al. "Triclosan-An Update." *Lett Appl Microbiol 52(2)* (Feb 2011):87–95.

[19] Jenkins, M. *What's Gotten into Us?: Staying Healthy in a Toxic World.* New York, NY: Random House, 2011.

[20] Pauling, L. *Vitamin C and the Common Cold.* San Francisco, CA: W.H. Freeman, 1970, 1976.

[21] Hickey, S., A.W. Saul. *Vitamin C: The Real Story, the Remarkable and Controversial*

Healing Factor. Laguna Beach, CA: Basic Health Publications, 2008.

[22] Lappé, F.M. *Diet for a Small Planet.* New York, NY: Ballantine Books, 1971.

[23] Hickey, S., H. Roberts. *Ascorbate: The Science of Vitamin C.* Morrisville, NC: Lulu.com, 2004.

[24] Levy, T.E. *Curing the Incurable: Vitamin C, Infectious Diseases, and Toxins.* Henderson, NV: LivOn Books, 2002. Levy, T.E. *Stop America's #1 Killer: Reversible Vitamin Deficiency Found to be Origin of All Coronary Heart Disease.* Henderson, NV: LivOn Books, 2006. Hickey, S., A.W. Saul. *Vitamin C: The Real Story, the Remarkable and Controversial Healing Factor.* Laguna Beach, CA: Basic Health Publications, 2008. Khalsa, S. *The Vitamin D Revolution: How the Power of This Amazing Vitamin Can Change Your Life.* Carlsbad, CA: Hay House, 2009. Holick, M.F. *The Vitamin D Solution: A 3-Step Strategy to Cure Our Most Common Health Problem.* New York, NY: Hudson Street Press, 2010.

[25] Dean, C. *The Magnesium Miracle.* New York, NY: Ballantine, 2007.

[26] Levy, T.E. *Curing the Incurable: Vitamin C, Infectious Diseases, and Toxins.* Henderson, NV: LivOn Books, 2002. Nahas, R., A. Balla. "Complementary and Alternative Medicine for Prevention and Treatment of the Common Cold." *Can Fam Physician* 57(1) (Jan 2011).

Uchide, N., H. Toyoda. "Antioxidant Therapy as a Potential Approach to Severe Influenza-Associated Complications." *Molecules* 16(3):(Feb 28, 2011):2032–2052.

[27] Levy, T.E. *Curing the Incurable: Vitamin C, Infectious Diseases, and Toxins.* Henderson, NV: LivOn Books, 2002. Hickey, S., A.W. Saul. *Vitamin C: The Real Story, the Remarkable and Controversial Healing Factor.* Laguna Beach, CA: Basic Health Publications, 2008.

[28] Levy, T.E. *Stop America's #1 Killer: Reversible Vitamin Deficiency Found to be Origin of All Coronary Heart Disease.* Henderson, NV: LivOn Books, 2006.

[29] Lien, E.L., B.R. Hammond. "Nutritional Influences on Visual Development and Function." *Prog Retin Eye Res* 30(3) (May 2011):188–203.

[30] Pauling, L. *How to Live Longer And Feel Better.* Corvallis, OR: Oregon State University Press, 1986, 2006. Hickey, S., A.W. Saul. *Vitamin C: The Real Story, the Remarkable and Controversial Healing Factor.* Laguna Beach, CA: Basic Health Publications, 2008.

[31] Maggini, S., E.S. Wintergerst, S. Beveridge, et al. "Selected Vitamins and Trace Elements Support Immune Function by Strengthening Epithelial Barriers and Cellular and Humoral Immune Responses." *Br J Nutr* 98 Suppl 1 (Oct 2007):S29–35.

[32] Pauling, L. *How to Live Longer And Feel Better.* Corvallis, OR: Oregon State University Press, 1986, 2006. Hickey, S., A.W. Saul. *Vitamin C: The Real Story, the Remarkable and Controversial Healing Factor.* Laguna Beach, CA: Basic Health Publications, 2008.

[33] Pauling, L. *How to Live Longer And Feel Better.* Corvallis, OR: Oregon State University Press, 1986, 2006. Johnson, R.J., E.A. Gaucher, Y.Y. Sautin, et al. "The Planetary Biology of Ascorbate and Uric Acid and Their Relationship with the Epidemic of Obesity and Cardiovascular Disease." *Med Hypotheses* 71(1) (2008):22–31.

[34] Pauling, L. *How to Live Longer And Feel Better.* Corvallis, OR: Oregon State University Press, 1986, 2006.

[35] Johnson, R.J., E.A. Gaucher, Y.Y. Sautin, et al. "The Planetary Biology of Ascorbate and Uric Acid and Their Relationship with the Epidemic of Obesity and Cardiovascular Disease." *Med Hypotheses* 71(1) (2008):22–31.

[36] Pauling, L. *How to Live Longer And Feel Better.* Corvallis, OR: Oregon State University Press, 1986, 2006.

[37] Ibid.

[38] Dean, C. *The Magnesium Miracle.* New York, NY: Ballantine, 2007.

[39] Levy, T.E. *Stop America's #1 Killer: Reversible Vitamin Deficiency Found to be Origin of All Coronary Heart Disease.* Henderson, NV: LivOn

Books, 2006. Hickey, S., A.W. Saul. *Vitamin C: The Real Story, the Remarkable and Controversial Healing Factor.* Laguna Beach, CA: Basic Health Publications, 2008.

[40] Lumey, L.H., A.D. Stein, E. Susser. "Prenatal Famine and Adult Health." *Annu Rev Public Health* 32 (Apr 21, 2011):237–2623.

[41] Ibid.

[42] Buecker, T.R. "Flour Milling in Nebraska." Nebraska State Historical Society, http://www.usgennet.org/usa/ne/topic/resources/NSHS/EDLFT/edlftl7.html. Tann, J., R.G.. Jones. "Technology and Transformation: The Diffusion of the Roller Mill in the British Flour Milling Industry, 1870-1907." *Technol Cult* 37(1) (Jan 1996):36–69. Also at: http://www.jstor.org/stable/3107201

[43] Funk, C. and H.E. Dubin. *The Vitamines.* Baltimore, MD: Williams and Wilkins Company, 1922.

[44] Fan, M.S., F.J. Zhao, S.J. Fairweather-Tait, et al. "Evidence of Decreasing Mineral Density in Wheat Grain Over the Last 160 Years." *J Trace Elem Med Biol* 22(4) (2008):315-324.

[45] Dean, C. *The Magnesium Miracle.* New York, NY: Ballantine, 2007. Thomas, D. "The Mineral Depletion of Foods Available to Us as a Nation (1940-2002)-a Review of the 6th Edition of McCance and Widdowson." *Nutr Health.* 19(1-2) (2007):21–55.

[46] Crinnion, W.J. "Organic Foods Contain Higher Levels of Certain Nutrients, Lower Levels of Pesticides and May Provide Health Benefits for the Consumer." *Altern Med Rev* 15(1) (Apr 2010):4–12.

[47] Beaton, G.H. "Recommended Dietary Intakes: Individuals and Populations." Chapter 103 in *Modern Nutrition in Health and Disease,* editors M.E. Shils, J.A. Olson, M. Shike, et al., 9th ed. Baltimore, MD: Williams & Wilkins, 1999.

[48] Holick, M.F. *The Vitamin D Solution: A 3-Step Strategy to Cure Our Most Common Health Problem.* New York, NY: Hudson Street Press, 2010.

[49] Hickey, S., A.W. Saul. *Vitamin C: The Real Story, the Remarkable and Controversial Healing Factor.* Laguna Beach, CA: Basic Health Publications, 2008.

[50] Ibid.

[51] Williams, R.J., G. Deason. "Individuality in Vitamin C Needs." *Proc Natl Acad Sci USA* 57(6) (Jun 1967):1638–1641.

[52] Elsas, L.J., P.B. Acosta. "Nutritional Support of Inherited Metabolic Diseases." Chapter 61 in *Modern Nutrition in Health and Disease,* editors M.E. Shils, J.A. Olson, M. Shike, et al., 9th ed. Baltimore, MD: Williams & Wilkins, 1999.

[53] Weir, D.G., J.M. Scott. "Vitamin B_{12} "Cobalamin"". Chapter 27 in *Modern Nutrition in Health and Disease,* editors M.E. Shils, J.A.

Olson, M. Shike, et al., 9th ed. Baltimore, MD: Williams & Wilkins, 1999. Pacholok, S.M., J.J. Stuart. *Could It Be B_{12}: An Epidemic of Misdiagnoses.* Sanger, CA: Quill Driver Books/Word Dancer Press, 2005.

[54] Montel-Hagen, A., M. Sitbon, N. Taylor. "Erythroid Glucose Transporters." *Curr Opin Hematol* 16(3) (May 2009):165–172.

[55] Stoyanovsky, D.A., R. Goldman, R.M. Darrow, et al. "Endogenous Ascorbate Regenerates Vitamin E in the Retina Directly and in Combination with Exogenous Dihydrolipoic Acid." *Curr Eye Res* 14(3) (Mar 1995):181–189. Papas, A. *The Vitamin E Factor: The Miraculous Antioxidant for the Prevention and Treatment of Heart disease, Cancer, and Aging.* New York, NY: HarperCollins, 1999.

[56] Violi, F. "Introduction to Nutraceuticals Special Issue." *Cardiovasc Ther* 28(4) (Aug 2010):185–186. Chakrabarti, S., J.E. Freedman. "Review: Nutriceuticals as Antithrombotic Agents." *Cardiovasc Ther* 28(4) (Aug 2010):227–235. Badimon, L., G. Vilahur, T. Padro. "Nutraceuticals and Atherosclerosis: Human Trials." *Cardiovasc Ther* 28(4) (Aug 2010):202–215. Davi, G., F. Santilli, C. Patrono. "Nutraceuticals in Diabetes and Metabolic Syndrome." *Cardiovasc Ther* 28(4) (Aug 2010):216–226. Zuchi, C., G. Ambrosio, T.F. Liischer, et al. "Nutraceuticals in Cardiovas-

cular Prevention: Lessons from Studies on Endothelial Function." *Cardiovasc Ther* 28(4) (Aug 2010):187–201.
[57] Grayson, M. "Nutrigenomics." *Nature* 468(7327) (Dec 23, 2010):S1.
[58] Laursen, L. "Interdisciplinary Research: Big Science at the Table." *Nature* 468(7327) (Dec 23, 2010):52–54.
[59] Stafford, N. "History: The Changing Notion of food." *Nature* 468(7327) (Dec 23, 2010):516–17.
[60] Frood, A. "Technology: A Flavour of the Future." *Nature* 468(7327) (Dec 23, 2010):S21–22.
[61] Pauling, L. "Orthomolecular Psychiatry." *Science* 160(825) (Apr 19, 1968):265–271. Pauling, L. *How to Live Longer And Feel Better.* Corvallis, OR: Oregon State University Press, 1986, 2006.
[62] Ausman, L.M., R.M. Russell "Nutrition in the Elderly." Chapter 53 in *Modern Nutrition in Health and Disease,* editors M.E. Shils, J.A. Olson, M. Shike, et al., 9th ed. Baltimore, MD: Williams & Wilkins, 1999.
[63] Keeley, E.C., B. Mehrad, R.M. Strieter. "Fibrocytes: Bringing New Insights into Mechanisms of Inflammation and Fibrosis." *Int J Biochem Cell Biol 42(4)* (Apr 2010):535–542.
[64] Ames, B.N. "Optimal Micronutrients Delay Mitochondrial Decay and Age-Associated Diseases."

Mech Ageing Dev 131 (2010):473–479. Selhub, J., A. Troen, I.H. Rosenberg. "B Vitamins and the Aging Brain." *Nutr Rev* 68(Suppl 2) (Dec 2010):S112–118.

[65] Ausman, L.M., R.M. Russell "Nutrition in the Elderly." Chapter 53 in *Modern Nutrition in Health and Disease,* editors M.E. Shils, J.A. Olson, M. Shike, et al., 9th ed. Baltimore, MD: Williams & Wilkins, 1999.

[66] Ames, B.N. "Low Micronutrient Intake May Accelerate the Degenerative Diseases of Aging through Allocation of Scarce Micronutrients by Triage." *Proc Natl Acad Sci USA.* 103 (2006):17589–17594. Dean, C. *The Magnesium Miracle.* New York, NY: Ballantine, 2007. Hoffer, A., A.W. Saul. *Orthomolecular Medicine for Everyone: Megavitamin Therapeutics for Families and Physicians.* Laguna Beach, CA: Basic Health Publications, 2008.

[67] Dean, C. *The Magnesium Miracle.* New York, NY: Ballantine, 2007.

[68] Ibid.

[69] Ames, B.N. "Low Micronutrient Intake May Accelerate the Degenerative Diseases of Aging through Allocation of Scarce Micronutrients by Triage." *Proc Natl Acad Sci USA.* 103 (2006):17589–17594.

[70] Ibid.

[71] Ibid.

[72] Ibid.

[73] Ames, B.N. "Optimal Micronutrients Delay Mitochondrial Decay and Age-Associated Diseases." *Mech Ageing Dev*131(2010):473–479.

[74] Selhub, J., et al. "B Vitamins and the Aging Brain." *Nutr Rev* 68(Suppl 2) (Dec 2010):S112–118. Manolescu, B.N., E. Oprea, I.C. Farcasanu, et al. "Homocysteine and Vitamin Therapy in Stroke Prevention and Treatment: a Review." *Acta Biochim Pol 57(4)* (2010):467477.

[75] Levy, T.E. *Stop America's #1 Killer: Reversible Vitamin Deficiency Found to be Origin of All Coronary Heart Disease.* Henderson, NV: LivOn Books, 2006.

Chapter 2. How Science Learns: Studies of Treatments

[76] Hickey, S., A.W. Saul. *Vitamin C: The Real Story, the Remarkable and Controversial Healing Factor.* Laguna Beach, CA: Basic Health Publications, 2008.

[77] Khalsa, S. *The Vitamin D Revolution: How the Power of This Amazing Vitamin Can Change Your Life.* Carlsbad, CA: Hay House, 2009. Holick, M.F. *The Vitamin D Solution: A 3-Step Strategy to Cure Our Most Common Health Problem.* New York, NY: Hudson Street Press, 2010.

[78] Zarbin, M.A., P.J. Rosenfeld. "Pathway-Based Therapies for Age-Related Macular Degeneration: an Integrated Survey of Emerging Treatment Alternatives." *Retina.* 30(9) (Oct 2010):1350–1367.

[79] Fine, L.C., J.S. Heier. *The Aging Eye: Preventing and Treating Eye Disease.* Special Health Reports. Boston, MA: Harvard Medical School, 2010.

[80] Cass, H. *Supplement Your Prescription: What Your Doctor Doesn't Know About Nutrition.* Launa Beach, CA: Basic Health Publications, 2007.

[81] Matthews, J.N.S. *Introduction to Randomized Controlled Clinical Trials,* 2nd Edition. Boca Raton, FL: Chapman & Hall/CRC, 2006.

[82] Berg, H.C. "Chemotaxis in Bacteria." *Annu Rev Biophys Bioeng* 4(1) (Jun 1 1975):119–136.

[83] Houston, M.C. "The Role of Cellular Micronutrient Analysis, Nutraceuticals, Vitamins, Antioxidants and Minerals in the Prevention and Treatment of Hypertension and Cardiovascular Disease." *Ther Adv Cardiovasc Dis* 4(3) (Jun 2010):165–183.

[84] Ames, B.N. "Low Micronutrient Intake May Accelerate the Degenerative Diseases of Aging through Allocation of Scarce Micronutrients by Triage." *Proc Natl Acad Sci USA.* 103 (2006):17589–17594.

[85] Ibid.

[86] West, A.L., G.A. Oren, S.E. Moroi. "Evidence for the Use of Nutritional Supplements and Herbal Medicines in Common Eye Diseases." *Am J Ophthalmol* 141(1) (Jan 2006):157–166

[87] Pauling, L. *How to Live Longer And Feel Better.* Corvallis, OR: Oregon State University Press, 1986, 2006.

[88] Simpson, S. Jr., B. Taylor, L. Blizzard, et al. "Higher 25-Hydroxyvitamin D is Associated with Lower Relapse Risk in Multiple Sclerosis." *Ann Neurol* 68(2) (Aug 2010):193-203. Urashima, M., T. Segawa, M. Okazaki, et al. "Randomized Trial of Vitamin D Supplementation to Prevent Seasonal Infuenza A in Schoolchildren." *Am J Clin Nutr* 91(5) (May 2010):1255–1260. Lucas, R.M., A.L. Ponsonby, K. Dear, et al. "Sun Exposure and Vitamin D Are Independent Risk Factors for CNS Demyelination." *Neurology* 76(6) (Feb 8 2011):540–548. Lucas, R.M., A.L. Ponsonby, K. Dear, et al. "Sun Exposure and Vitamin D Are Independent Risk Factors for CNS Demyelination." *Neurology* 76(6) (Feb 8 2011):540–548.

[89] Parekh, N., R.J. Chappell, A.E. Millen, et al. "Association Between Vitamin D and Age-Related Macular Degeneration in the Third National Health and Nutrition Examination Survey, 1988 through 1994." *Arch Ophthalmol* 125(5) (May 2007):661–669. Mascitelli, L., F. Pezzetta, M.R. Goldstein. "Macular Degeneration, Heart Dis-

ease, and Vitamin D." *Ophthalmology.* 117(1) (Jan 2010):194.

[90] de Jong, P.T. "Age-Related Macular Degeneration." *N Engl J Med* 355(14) (Oct 5, 2006):1474–1485.

Chapter 3. The Eye: How It Works, and What Can Go Wrong

[91] Rodieck, R.W. *The First Steps in Seeing.* Sunderland, MA: Sinauer, 1998.

[92] Ibid.

[93] Ibid.

[94] Curcio, C.A., K.R. Sloan, R.E. Kalina, et al. "Human Photoreceptor Topography." *J Comp Neurol* 292(4) (1990):497–523.

[95] Strauss, O. "The Retinal Pigment Epithelium in Visual Function." *Physiol Rev* 85(3) (2005):845–881.

[96] Runkle, E.A., D.A. Antonetti. "The Blood-Retinal Barrier: Structure and Functional Significance." *Methods Mol Biol*686(2011):133–148.

[97] Ibid.

[98] Thomas, J.A. "Oxidative Stress and Oxidant Defense." Chapter 46 in *Modern Nutrition in Health and Disease,* editors M.E. Shils, J.A. Olson, M. Shike, et al., 9th ed. Baltimore, MD: Williams & Wilkins, 1999. Finkel, T., N.J. Holbrook. "Oxidants, Oxidative Stress and the Biology of Ageing." *Nature* 408(6809) (Nov 9,

2000):239–247. Mozaffarieh, M., J. Flammer. "A Novel Perspective on Natural Therapeutic Approaches in Glaucoma Therapy." *Expert Opin Emerging Drugs* 12(2) (May 2007):195–198.

[99] International Agency for Research on Cancer. *IARC Monographs on the Evaluation of Carcinogenic Risks to Humans: Tobacco Smoke and Involuntary Smoking.* Volume 83 (2004). Available from http://www.iarc.fr.

[100] Finaud, J., G.. Lac, E. Filaire. "Oxidative Stress: Relationship with Exercise and Training." *Sports Med* 36(4) (2006):327–358. Pashkow, F.J., D.G. Watumull, C.L. Campbell. "Astaxanthin: a Novel Potential Treatment for Oxidative Stress and Inflammation in Cardiovascular Disease." *Am J Cardiol* 101(10A) (May 22, 2008):58D-68D. Farbstein, D., A. Kozak-Blickstein, A.P. Levy. "Antioxidant Vitamins and Their Use in Preventing Cardiovascular Disease." *Molecules* 15(11) (2010):8098–8110. Yfanti, C., A.R. Nielsen, T.C. Akerstrom, et al. "The Effect of Antioxidant Supplementation on Insulin-Sensitivity in Response to Endurance Exercise Training." *Am J Physiol Endocrinol Metab* 300(5) (May 201 1):E761–770.

[101] Hickey, S., A.W. Saul. *Vitamin C: The Real Story, the Remarkable and Controversial*

Healing Factor. Laguna Beach, CA: Basic Health Publications, 2008.

[102] Reiss, G.. R., P.G. Werness, P.E. Zollman, et al. "Ascorbic Acid Levels in the Aqueous Humor of Nocturnal and Diurnal Mammals." *Arch Ophthalmol* 104(5) (May 1986):753–755. Gross, R.L. "Collagen Type I and III Synthesis by Tenon's Capsule Fibroblasts in Culture: Individual Patient Characteristics and Response to Mitomycin C, 5-Fluo-rouracil, and Ascorbic Acid." *Trans Am Ophthalmol Soc 97* (1999):513–543.

[103] Stoyanovsky, D.A., R. Goldman, R.M. Darrow, et al. "Endogenous Ascorbate Regenerates Vitamin E in the Retina Directly and in Combination with Exogenous Dihydrolipoic Acid." *Curr Eye Res* 14(3) (Mar 1995):181–189. Jacob, R.A. "Vitamin C." Chapter 29 in *Modern Nutrition in Health and Disease,* editors M.E. Shils, J.A. Olson, M. Shike, et al., 9th ed. Baltimore, MD: Williams & Wilkins, 1999.

[104] Finkel, T., N.J. Holbrook. "Oxidants, Oxidative Stress and the Biology of Ageing." *Nature* 408(6809) (Nov 9, 2000):239–247.

[105] Azzi, A. "Molecular Mechanism of Alpha-Tocopherol Action." *Free Radic Biol Med* 43(1) (July 1, 2007):16–21. Engin, K.N. "Alpha-Tocopherol: Looking Beyond an Antioxidant." *Mol Vis* 15 (2009):855–860. Traber,

M.G. "Regulation of Xenobiotic Metabolism, the Only Signaling Function of Alpha-Tocopherol?" *Mol Nutr Food Res* 54(5) (May 2010):661–668.

[106] Young, R.W. "The Family of Sunlight-Related Eye Diseases." *Optom Vis Sci* 71(2) (Feb 1994):125–144. Tezel, G.. "Oxidative Stress in Glaucomatous Neurodegeneration: Mechanisms and Consequences." *Prog Retin Eye* Res 25(5) (Sep 2006):490–513. Williams, D. L, "Oxidation, Antioxidants and Cataract Formation: A Literature Review." *Vet Ophthalmol* 9(5) (Sep-Oct 2006):292–298. Williams, D. L. "Oxidative Stress and the Eye." *Vet Clin North Am Small Anim Pract* 38(1) (Jan 2008):179–192, vii.

[107] Bouton, S.M., Jr. "Vitamin C and the Aging Eye. An Experimental Clinical Study." *Arch Intern Med* 63(5) (1939):930–945.

[108] Rhone, M., A. Basu. "Phytochemicals and Age-Related Eye Diseases." *Nutr Rev* 66(8) (Aug 2008):465–472.

[109] Maritim, A.C., R.A. Sanders, J.B. Watkins III. "Diabetes, Oxidative Stress, and Antioxidants: A Review." *J Biochem Mol Toxicol* 17(1) (2003):24–38.

[110] Ames, B.N. "Optimal Micronutrients Delay Mitochondrial Decay and Age-associated Diseases." *Mech Ageing Dev* 131 (2010):473–479.

[111] Lien, E.L., B.R. Hammond. "Nutritional Influences on Visual Development and Function." *Prog Retin Eye Res* 30(3) (May 2011):188203.

[112] Sasaki, M., K. Yuki, T. Kurihara, et al. "Biological Role of Lutein in the Light-Induced Retinal Degeneration." *J Nutr Biochem* (Jun 8 2011) Epub ahead of print. http://www.ncbi.nlm.nih.gov/pubmed/21658930.

[113] Rhone, M., A. Basu. "Phytochemicals and Age-Related Eye Diseases." *Nutr Rev* 66(8) (Aug 2008):465–472. Sasaki, M., K. Yuki, T. Kurihara, et al. "Biological Role of Lutein in the Light-Induced Retinal Degeneration." *J Nutr Biochem* (Jun 8, 2011) Epub ahead of print http://www.ncbi.nlm.nih.gov/pubmed/21658930.

[114] Handelman. G.J., E.A. Dratz, C.C. Reay, et al. "Carotenoids in the Human Macula and Whole Retina." *Invest Ophthalmol Vis Sci* 29(6, (Jun 1988):850–855.

[115] Lien, E.L., B.R. Hammond. "Nutritional Influences on Visual Development and Function." *Prog Retin Eye Res* 30(3) (May 2011):188–203.

[116] Terrasa, A.M., M.H. Guajardo, C.A. Marra, et al. "Alpha-Tocopherol Protects Against Oxidative Damage to Lipids of the Rod Outer Segments of the Equine Retina." *Vet J* 182(3) (Dec 2009):463–468.

[117] Veach, J. "Functional Dichotomy: Glutathione and Vitamin E in Homeostasis Relevant to Primary Open-Angle Glaucoma." *Br J Nutr* 91(6) (Jun 2004):809–829.

[118] Stoyanovsky, D.A., R. Goldman, R.M. Darrow, et al. "Endogenous Ascorbate Regenerates Vitamin E in the Retina Directly and in Combination with Exogenous Dihydrolipoic Acid." *Curr Eye Res* 14(3) (Mar 1995):181–189.

[119] Skulachev, V.P. "New Data on Biochemical Mechanism of Programmed Senescence of Organisms and Antioxidant Defense of Mitochondria." *Biochemistry (Mosc)* 74(12) (Dec 2009):1400–1403.

[120] Skulachev, V.P. "New Data on Biochemical Mechanism of Programmed Senescence of Organisms and Antioxidant Defense of Mitochondria." *Biochemistry (Mosc)* 74(12) (Dec 2009):1400–1403. Jin, H.X., J. Randazzo, P. Zhang, et al. "Multifunctional Antioxidants for the Treatment of Age-Related Diseases." *J Med Chem* 53(3) (Feb 11, 2010):1117–1127.

Chapter 4. The Effects of Light on the Eye

[121] Young, R.W. "The Family of Sunlight-Related Eye Diseases." *Optom Vis Sci* 71(2) (Feb 1994):125–144.

[122] Khalsa, S. *The Vitamin D Revolution: How the Power of This Amazing Vitamin Can Change Your Life.* Carlsbad, CA: Hay House, 2009. Holick, M.F. *The Vitamin D Solution: A 3-Step Strategy to Cure Our Most Common Health Problem.* New York, NY: Hud-son Street Press, 2010 Dowdy, J.C., R.M. Sayre, M.F. Holick "Holick's Rule and Vitamin D from Sunlight." *J Steroid Biochem Mol Biol* 121(1-2) (Jul 2010):328–330.

[123] Young, R.W. "The Family of Sunlight-Related Eye Diseases." *Optom Vis Sci* 71(2) (Feb 1994):125–144.

[124] Tezel, G. "Oxidative Stress in Glaucomatous Neurodegeneration: Mechanisms and Consequences." *Prog Retin Eye Res* 25(5) (Sep 2006):490–513. Skulachev, V.P., Anisimov, V.N., Antonenko, Y.N., et al. "An Attempt to Prevent Senescence: A Mitochondrial Approach." *Biochim Biophys Acta* 1787(5) (May 2009):437–461.

[125] Beatty, S., H. Koh, M. Phil, D. Henson, et al. "The Role of Oxidative Stress in the

Pathogenesis of Age-Related Macular Degeneration." *Surv Ophthalmol 45(2)* (Sep-Oct 2000):115–134.

[126] Finkel, T., N.J. Holbrook. "Oxidants, Oxidative Stress and the Biology of Ageing." *Nature* 408(6809) (Nov 9, 2000):239–247. Tezel, G.. "Oxidative Stress in Glaucomatous Neurodegeneration: Mechanisms and Consequences." *Prog Retin Eye* Res 25(5) (Sep 2006):490–513. Osborne, N.N., G.Y. Li, D. Ji, et al. "Light Affects Mitochondria to Cause Apoptosis to Cultured Cells: Possible Relevance to Ganglion Cell Death in Certain Optic Neuropathies." *J Neurochem* 105(5) (Jun 2008):2013–2028.

[127] Young, R.W. "The Renewal of Rod and Cone Outer Segments in the Rhesus Monkey." *J Cell Biol 49(2)* (May 1, 1971):303–318.

[128] Rodieck, R.W. *The First Steps in Seeing.* Sunderland, MA: Sinauer, 1998.

[129] Organisciak, D.T., D.K. Vaughan. "Retinal Light Damage: Mechanisms and Protection." *Prog Retin Eye* Res 29(2) (Mar 2010):113–134.

[130] Noell, W.K. "Effects of Environmental Lighting and Dietary Vitamin A on the Vulnerability of the Retina to Light Damage." *Photochem Photobiol* 29(4) (Apr 1979):717–723.

[131] Organisciak, D.T., H.M. Wang, Z.Y. Li, et al. "The Protective Effect of Ascorbate in Retinal

Light Damage of Rats." *Invest Ophthalmol Vis Sci* 26(11) (Nov 1985):1580–1588.

[132] Organisciak, D.T., I.R. Bicknell, R.M. Darrow. "The Effects of L-and D-Ascorbic Acid Administration on Retinal Tissue Levels and Light Damage in Rats." *Curr Eye Res* 11(3) (Mar 1992):231–241.

[133] Tanito, M., A. Nishiyama, T. Tanaka, et al. "Change of Redox Status and Modulation by Thiol Replenishment in Retinal Photooxidative Damage." *Invest Ophthalmol Vis Sci* 43(7) (Jul 2002):2392–2400.

[134] Organisciak, D.T., D.K. Vaughan. "Retinal Light Damage: Mechanisms and Protection." *Prog Retin Eye* Res 29(2) (Mar 2010):113–134.

[135] Ibid.

[136] Hickey, S., A.W. Saul. *Vitamin C: The Real Story, the Remarkable and Controversial Healing Factor.* Laguna Beach, CA: Basic Health Publications, 2008.

[137] Rodieck, R.W. *The First Steps in Seeing.* Sunderland, MA: Sinauer, 1998.

[138] Linton, J.D., L.C. Holzhausen, N. Babai, et al. "Flow of Energy in the Outer Retina in Darkness and in Light." *Proc Natl Acad Sci USA* 107(19) (May 2010):8599–8604.

[139] Young, R.W. "The Family of Sunlight-Related Eye Diseases." *Optom Vis Sci* 71(2) (Feb 1994):125–144.

[140] Fernandez, M.M., N.A. Afshari. "Cataracts: We Have Perfected the Surgery, But Is It Time for Prevention?" *Curr Opin Ophthalmol* 22(1) (Jan 2011):2–3.

[141] Rafnsson, V., E. Olafsdottir, J. Hrafnkelsson, et al. "Cosmic Radiation Increases the Risk of Nuclear Cataract in Airline Pilots: A Population-Based Case-Control Study." *Arch Ophthalmol* 123(8) (Aug 2005):1102–1105.

[142] Hiller, R., R.D. Sperduto, M.J. Podgor, et al. "Cigarette Smoking and the Risk of Development of Lens Opacities. The Framingham Studies." *Arch Ophthalmol* 115(9) (Sep 1997):1113–1118. Mares, J.A., R. Voland, R. Adler R, et al.; CAREDS Group. "Healthy Diets and the Subsequent Prevalence of Nuclear Cataract in Women." *Arch Ophthalmol* 128(6) (Jun 2010):738–749.

[143] Handelman, G.J., L. Packer, C.E. Cross. "Destruction of Tocopherols, Carotenoids, and Retinol in Human Plasma by Cigarette Smoke." *Am J Clin Nutr* 63 (1996):559–565. Frikke-Schmidt, H., P. Tveden-Nyborg, M.M. Birck, et al. "High Dietary Fat and Cholesterol Exacerbates Chronic Vitamin C Deficiency in Guinea Pigs." *Br J Nutr* 105(1) (Jan 2011):54–61.

[144] Mosad, S.M., A.A. Ghanem, H.M. El-Fallal, et al. "Lens Cadmium, Lead, and Serum Vitamins C, E, and Beta Carotene in Cataractous

Smoking Patients." *Curr Eye Res* 35(1) (Jan 2010):23–30.

[145] Williams, D.L. "Oxidation, Antioxidants and Cataract Formation: A Literature Review." *Vet Ophthalmol* 9(5) (Sep-Oct 2006):292–298. Mares, J.A., R. Voland, R. Adler R, et al.; CAREDS Group. "Healthy Diets and the Subsequent Prevalence of Nuclear Cataract in Women." *Arch Ophthalmol* 128(6) (Jun 2010):738–749.

[146] Ma, L., X.M. Lin. "Effects of Lutein and Zeaxanthin on Aspects of Eye Health." *J Sci Food Agric* 90(1) (Jan 2010):2–12.

[147] Rouhiainen, P., H. Rouhiainen, J.T. Salonen. "Association Between Low Plasma Vitamin E Concentration and Progression of Early Cortical Lens Opacities." *Am J Epidemiol* 144(5) (Sep 1, 1996):496–500. Nourmohammadi, I., M. Modarress, K. Khanaki, et al. "Association of Serum Alpha-Tocopherol, Retinol and Ascorbic Acid with the Risk of Cataract Development." *Ann Nutr Metab* 52(4) (2008):296–298. Engin, K.N. "Alpha-Tocopherol: Looking Beyond an Antioxidant." *Mol Vis* 15 (2009):855–860.

[148] Packer, L. "Protective Role of Vitamin E in Biological Systems." *Am J Clin Nutr* 53 (1991):10505–10555. Seth, R.K., S. Kharb. "Protective Function of Alpha-Tocopherol Against the Process of Cataractogenesis in

Humans." *Ann Nutr Metab.* 43(5) (1999):286–289. Lyle, B.J., J.A. Mares-Perlman, B.E. Klein, et al. "Serum Carotenoids and Tocopherols and Incidence of Age-Related Nuclear Cataract." *Am J Clin Nutt* 69 (2) (Feb 1999):272–277. Head, K.A. "Natural Therapies for Ocular Disorders, Part Two: Cataracts and Glaucoma." *Altern Med Rev 6(2)* (Apr 2001):141–166. Rhone, M., A. Basu. "Phytochemicals and Age-Related Eye Diseases." *Nutr Rev* 66(8) (Aug 2008):465–472.

[149] Jacques, P.F., A. Taylor, S.E. Hankinson, et al. "Long-Term Vitamin C Supplement Use and Prevalence of Early Age-Related Opacities." *Am J Clin Nutr* 66(4) (Oct 1997):911–916. Head, K.A. "Natural Therapies for Ocular Disorders, Part Two: Cataracts and Glaucoma." *Altcrn Med Rev* 6(2) (Apr 2001):141–166. Fernandez, M.M., N.A. Afshari. "Cataracts: We Have Perfected the Surgery, But Is It Time for Prevention?" *Curr Opin Ophthalmol 22(1)* (Jan 2011):2–3.

[150] Christen, W.G., R.J. Glynn, H.D. Sesso, et al. "Age-Related Cataract in a Randomized Trial of Vitamins E and C in Men." *Arch Ophthalmol* 128(11) (Nov 2010):1397–1405.

[151] Ibid.

[152] Papas, A. *The Vitamin E Factor: The Miraculous Antioxidant for the Prevention and*

Treatment of Heart disease, Cancer, and Aging. New York, NY: HarperCollins, 1999.

[153] Papas, A. *The Vitamin E Factor: The Miraculous Antioxidant for the Prevention and Treatment of Heart disease, Cancer, and Aging.* New York, NY: HarperCollins, 1999. Jensen, S.K., C. Lauridsen. "Alpha-Tocopherol Stereo isomers." *Vitam Horm* 76 (2007):281–308.

[154] Hoffer, A., A.W. Saul. *Orthomolecular Medicine for Everyone: Megavitamin Therapeutics for Families and Physicians.* Laguna Beach. CA: Basic Health Publications, 2008.

[155] Jacob, R.A. "Vitamin C." Chapter 29 in *Modern Nutrition in Health and Disease,* editors M.E. Shils, J.A. Olson, M. Shike, et al., 9th ed Baltimore, MD: Williams & Wilkins, 1999. Hickey, S., A.W. Saul. *Vitamin C: The Real Story, the Remarkable and Controversial Healing Factor.* Laguna Beach, CA: Basic Health Publications, 2008.

[156] Hickey, S., A.W. Saul. *Vitamin C: The Real Story, the Remarkable and Controversial Healing Factor.* Laguna Beach, CA: Basic Health Publications, 2008.

[157] Head, K.A. "Natural Therapies for Ocular Disorders, Part Two: Cataracts and Glaucoma." *Altern Med Rev* 6(2) (Apr 2001):141–166.

[158] Ledesma, M.C., B. Jung-Hynes, T.L. Schmit, et al. "Selenium and Vitamin E for Prostate Cancer: Post-SELECT Status." *Mol Med* 17(1-2) (Jan-Feb 2011):134–143.

[159] Hegde, K.R., S.D. Varma. "Combination of Glycemic and Oxidative Stress in Lens: Implications in Augmentation of Cataract Formation in Diabetes." *Free Radic Res* 39(5) (May 2005):513–517.

[160] Wong, I.Y., S.C. Koo, C.W. Chan. "Prevention of Age-Related Macular Degeneration." *Int Ophthalmol* 31(1) (Feb 2011):73–82.

Chapter 5. Vitamins Prevent Degeneration of the Photoreceptors: Retinal Detachment, Macular Degeneration and Retinitis Pigmentosa

[161] Abouzeid, H., T.J. Wolfensberger. "Macular Recovery After Retinal Detachment." *Acta Ophthalmol Scand* 84(5) (Oct 2006):597–605.

[162] Marc, R.E., B.W. Jones, C.B. Watt, et al. "Extreme Retinal Remodeling Triggered by Light Damage: Implications for Age-Related Macular Degeneration." *Mol Vis* 14 (Apr 25, 2008):782–806.

[163] Wickham, L., D.G. Charteris. "Glial Cell Changes of the Human Retina in Proliferative

Vitreoretinopathy." *Dev Ophthalmol 44* (2009):37–45.

[164] Bohmer, J.A., B. Sellhaus, N.F. Schrage. "Effects of Ascorbic Acid on Retinal Pigment Epithelial Cells." *Curr Eye Res* 23(3) (Sep 2001):206–214.

[165] Gerona, G., D. Lopez, M. Palmero, et al. "Antioxidant N-Acetyl-Cysteine Protects Retinal Pigmented Epithelial Cells from Long-Term Hypoxia Changes in Gene Expression." *J Ocul Pharmacol Ther 26(4)* (Aug 2010):309–314.

[166] Bhooma, V., K.N. Sulochana, J. Biswas, et al. "E ales' Disease: Accumulation of Reactive Oxygen Intermediates and Lipid Peroxides and Decrease of Antioxidants Causing Inflammation, Neovascularization and Retinal Damage." *Curr Eye Res* 16(2) (Feb 1997):91–95.

[167] de Jong, P.T. "Age-Related Macular Degeneration." *N Engl J Med* 355(14) (Oct 5, 2006):1474–1485.

[168] Bertram, K.M., C.J. Baglole, R.P. Phipps, et al. "Molecular Regulation of Cigarette Smoke Induced-Oxidative Stress in Human Retinal Pigment Epithelial Cells: Implications for Age-Related Macular Degeneration." *Am J Physiol Cell Physiol* 297(5) (Nov 2009):C1200–1210.

[169] Beatty, S., H. Koh, M. Phil, D. Henson, et al. "The Role of Oxidative Stress in the Pathogenesis of Age-Related Macular Degeneration."

Surv Ophthalmol 45(2) (Sep-Oct 2000):115–134.

[170] de Jong, P.T. "Age-Related Macular Degeneration." *N Engl J Med* 355(14) (Oct 5, 2006):1474–1485. Bertram, K.M., C.J. Baglole, R.P. Phipps, et al. "Molecular Regulation of Cigarette Smoke Induced-Oxidative Stress in Human Retinal Pigment Epithelial Cells: Implications for Age-Related Macular Degeneration." *Am J Physiol Cell Physiol* 297(5) (Nov 2009):C1200–1210.

[171] Paetkau, M.E., T.A. Boyd, M. Grace, et al. "Senile Disciform Macular Degeneration and Smoking." *Can J Ophthalmol* 13(2) (Apr 1978):67–71.

[172] Evans, J.R., A.E. Fletcher, R.P. Wormald. "28,000 Cases of Age Related Macular Degeneration Causing Visual Loss in People Aged 75 Years and Above in the United Kingdom May Be Attributable to Smoking." *Br J Ophthalmol* 89(5) (May 2005):550–553. de Jong, P.T. "Age-Related Macular Degeneration. *N Engl J Med* 355(14) (Oct 5, 2006):1474–1485.

[173] Vardavas, C.I., D.B. Panagiotakos. "The Causal Relationship Between Passive Smoking and Inflammation on the Development of Cardiovascular Disease: A Review of the Evidence." *Inflamm Allergy Drug Targets* 8(5) (Dec 2009):328–333.

[174] Tan, J.S., P. Mitchell, A. Kifley, et al. "Smoking and the Long-Term Incidence of Age-Related Macular Degeneration: the Blue Mountains Eye Study." *Arch Ophthalmol* 125(8) (Aug 2007):1089–1095.

[175] Bertram, K.M., C.J. Baglole, R.P. Phipps, et al. "Molecular Regulation of Cigarette Smoke Induced-Oxidative Stress in Human Retinal Pigment Epithelial Cells: Implications for Age-Related Macular Degeneration." *Am J Physiol Cell Physiol* 297(5) (Nov 2009):C1200–1210.

[176] Ibid.

[177] Klein, R., T. Peto, A. Bird, et al. "The Epidemiology of Age-Related Macular Degeneration." *Am J Ophthalmol* 137(3) (Mar 2004):486495.

[178] de Jong, P.T. "Age-Related Macular Degeneration." *N Engl J Med* 355(14) (Oct 5, 2006):1474–1485. Fletcher, A.E., G.C. Bentham, M. Agnew, et al. "Sunlight Exposure, Antioxidants, and Age-Related Macular Degeneration." *Arch Ophthalmol* 126(10) (Oct 2008):1396–1403.

[179] Hageman, G.S., P.j. Luthert, N.H. Victor Chong, et al. "An Integrated Hypothesis That Considers Drusen as Biomarkers of Immune-Mediated Processes at the RPE-Bruchs Membrane Interface in Aging and Age-Related Macular Degeneration." *Prog Retin Eye Res* 20(6) (Nov 2001):705–732.

[180] de Jong, P.T. "Age-Related Macular Degeneration." *N Engl J Med* 355(14) (Oct 5, 2006):1474–1485.

[181] Lien, E.L., B.R. Hammond. "Nutritional Influences on Visual Development and Function." *Prog Retin Eye Res* 30(3) (May 2011):188203.

[182] Curcio, C.A., C.L. Millican, K.A. Allen, et al. "Aging of the Human Photoreceptor Mosaic: Evidence for Selective Vulnerability of Rods in Central Retina." *Invest Ophthalmol Vis Sci* 34(12) (Nov 1993):3278–3296.

[183] de Jong, P.T. "Age-Related Macular Degeneration." *N Engl J Med* 355(14) (Oct 5, 2006):1474–1485.

[184] Karunadharma, P.P., C.L. Nordgaard, T.W. Olsen, et al. "Mitochondrial DNA Damage as a Potential Mechanism for Age-related Macular Degeneration." *Invest Ophthalmol Vis Sci* 51(11) (Nov 2010):5470–5479.

[185] de Jong, P.T. "Age-Related Macular Degeneration." *N Engl J Med* 355(14) (Oct 5, 2006):1474–1485.

[186] Marc, R.E., B.W. Jones, C.B. Watt, et al. "Extreme Retinal Remodeling Triggered by Light Damage: Implications for Age Related Macular Degeneration." *Mol Vis* 14 (Apr 25, 2008):782–806.

[187] de Jong, P.T. "Age-Related Macular Degeneration." *N Engl J Med* 355(14) (Oct 5, 2006):1474–1485.

[188] AREDS, Age-Related Eye Disease Study Research Group. "A Randomized, Placebo-Controlled, Clinical Trial of High-Dose Supplementation with Vitamins C and E, Beta Carotene, and Zinc for Age-Related Macular Degeneration and Vision Loss: AREDS Report No. *8." Arch Ophthalmol* 119 (10) (Oct 2001):1417–1436. van Leeuwen, R., S. Boekhoorn, J.R. Vingerling, et al. "Dietary Intake of Antioxidants and Risk of Age-Related Macular Degeneration." *JAMA* 294(24) (Dec 28, 2005):3101–3107. Tan, J.S., J.J. Wang, V. Flood, et al. "Dietary Antioxidants and the Long-Term Incidence of Age-Related Macular Degeneration: The Blue Mountains Eye Study." *Ophthalmology* 115(2) (Feb 2008):334–341. Chiu, C.J., R.C. Milton, R. Klein, et al. "Dietary Compound Score and Risk of Age-Related Macular Degeneration in the Age-Related Eye Disease Study." *Ophthalmology* 116(5) (May 2009):939–946.

[189] AREDS, Age-Related Eye Disease Study Research Group. "A Randomized, Placebo-Controlled, Clinical Trial of High-Dose Supplementation with Vitamins C and E, Beta Carotene, and Zinc for Age-Related

Macular Degeneration and Vision Loss: AREDS Report No.8." *Arch Ophthalmol* 119(10) (Oct 2001):1417–1436.

[190] Chiu, C.J., R.C. Milton, R. Klein, et al. "Dietary Compound Score and Risk of Age-Related Macular Degeneration in the Age-Related Eye Disease Study." *Ophthalmology* 116(5) (May 2009):939–946.

[191] Johnson, E.J. "Age-Related Macular Degeneration and Antioxidant Vitamins: Recent Findings." *Curr Opin Clin Nutr Metab Care* 13(1) (Jan 2010):28–33

[192] Augood, C., U. Chakravarthy, I. Young, et al. "Oily Fish Consumption, Dietary Docosahexaenoic Acid and Eicosapentaenoic Acid Intakes, and Associations with Neovas-cular Age-Related Macular Degeneration." *Am J Clin Nutr 88(2)* (Aug 2008):398–406.

[193] Organisciak, D.T., D.K. Vaughan. "Retinal Light Damage: Mechanisms and Protection." *Prog Retin Eye Res* 29(2) (Mar 2010):113–134.

[194] SanGiovanni, J.P., E.Y. Chew. "The Role of Omega-3 Long-Chain Polyunsaturated Fatty Acids in Health and Disease of the Retina." *Prog Retin Eye Res* 24(1) (Jan 2005):87–138. SanGiovanni, J.P., E.Y. Chew, E. Agron, et al. "The Relationship of Dietary Omega-3 Long-Chain Polyunsaturated Fatty Acid Intake with Incident Age-Related Macular Degeneration:

AREDS Report No.23." *Arch Ophthalmol* 126 (9) (Sep 2008):1274–1279.

[195] Johnson, E.J. "Age-Related Macular Degeneration and Antioxidant Vitamins: Recent Findings." *Curr Opin Clin Nutr Metab Care* 13(1) (Jan 2010):28–33

[196] Christen, W.G., R.J. Glynn, E.Y. Chew, et al. "Folic Acid, Pyridoxine, and Cyanocobalamin Combination Treatment and Age-Related Macular Degeneration in Women: The Women's Antioxidant and Folic Acid Cardiovascular Study." *Arch Intern Med* 169(4) (Feb 23; 2009):335–341.

[197] Ibid.

[198] Manolescu, B.N., E. Oprea, I.C. Farcasanu, et al. "Homocysteine and Vitamin Therapy in Stroke Prevention and Treatment: a Review." *Acta Biochim Pol* 57(4) (2010):467–477.

[199] Selhub, J., A. Troen, I.H. Rosenberg. "B Vitamins and the Aging Brain." *Nutr Rev* 68(Suppl 2) (Dec 2010):S112–118.

[200] Christen, W.G., R.J. Glynn, E.Y. Chew, et al. "Folic Acid, Pyridoxine, and Cyanocobalamin Combination Treatment and Age-Related Macular Degeneration in Women: The Women's Antioxidant and Folic Acid Cardiovascular Study." *Arch Intern Med* 169(4) (Feb 23. 2009):335–341.

[201] Kaushik, S., J.J. Wang, V. Flood, et al. "Dietary Glycemic Index and the Risk of Age-

Related Macular Degeneration." *Am J Clin Nutt* 88 (4) (Oct 2008):1104–1110. Chiu, C.J., A. Taylor. "Dietary Hyperglycemia, Glycemic Index and Metabolic Retinal Diseases." *Prog Retin Eye Res* 30(1) (Jan 2011):18–53.

[202] Hu, Y., G. Block, E.P. Norkus, et al. "Relations of Glycemic Index and Glycemic Load with Plasma Oxidative Stress Markers." *Am J Clir Nutr* 84(1) (Jul 2006):70-76.

[203] Ledesma, M.C., B. Jung-Hynes, T.L. Schmit, et al. "Selenium and Vitamin E for Prostate Cancer: Post-SELECT Status." *Mol Med* 17(1-2) (Jan-Feb 2011):134–143.

[204] Johnson, E.J. "Age-Related Macular Degeneration and Antioxidant Vitamins: Recent Findings." *Curr Opin Clin Nutr Metab Care* 13(1) (Jan 2010):28–33. Pemp, B., F. Polska, K. Karl, et al. "Effects of Antioxidants (AREDS Medication) on Ocular Blood Flow and Endothelial Function in an Endotoxin-Induced Model of Oxidative Stress in Humans." *Invest Ophthalmol Vis Sci* 51(1) (Jan 2010):2–6.

[205] Christen, W.G., R.J. Glynn, E.Y. Chew, et al. "Vitamin E and Age-Related Macular Degeneration in a Randomized Trial of Women." *Ophthalmology* 117(6) (Jun 2010):1163–1168.

[206] Raniga, A., M.J. Elder. "Dietary Supplement Use in the Prevention of Age-Related Macular

Degeneration Progression." *NZ Med I* 122(1299) (Jul 24 2009):32–38.

[207] Parekh, N., R.J. Chappell, A.E. Millen, et al. "Association Between Vitamin D and Age-Related Macular Degeneration in the Third National Health and Nutrition Examination Survey, 1988 through 1994." *Arch Ophthalmol* 125(5) (May 2007):661–669. Mascitelli, L., F. Pezzetta, M.R. Goldstein. "Macular Degeneration, Heart Disease, and Vitamin D." *Ophthalmology.* 117(1) (Jan 2010):194.

[208] Maggini, S., E.S. Wintergerst, S. Beveridge, et al. "Selected Vitamins and Trace Elements Support Immune Function by Strengthening Epithelial Barriers and Cellular and Humoral Immune Responses." *Br J Nutr* 98 Suppl 1 (Oct 2007):529–35. Parekh, N., R.J. Chappell, A.E. Millen, et al. "Association Between Vitamin D and Age-Related Macular Degeneration in the Third National Health and Nutrition Examination Survey, 1988 through 1994." *Arch Ophthalmol* 125(5) (May 2007):661–669.

[209] Sun, C., R. Klein, T.Y. Wong. "Age-Related Macular Degeneration and Risk of Coronary Heart Disease and Stroke: The Cardiovascular Health Study." *Ophthalmology* 116(10) (Oct 2009):1913–1919.

[210] Mascitelli, L., F. Pezzetta, M.R. Goldstein. "Macular Degeneration, Heart Disease, and

Vitamin D." *Ophthalmology.*117(1)(Jan 2010):194.

[211] Organisciak, D.T., D.K. Vaughan. "Retinal Light Damage: Mechanisms and Protection." *Prog Retin Eye Res* 29(2) (Mar 2010):113–134.

[212] Lin, M.H., M.C. Wu, S. Lu, et al. "Glycemic Index, Glycemic Load and Insuline-mic Index of Chinese Starchy Foods." *World J Gastroenterol* 16(39) (Oct 21, 2010):4973–4979.

[213] Whelan, W.J., D. Hollar, A. Agatston, et al. "The Glycemic Response is a Personal Attribute." *IUBMB Life* 62(8) (Aug 2010):637–641.

[214] Richer, S., W. Stiles, C. Thomas. "Molecular Medicine in Ophthalmic Care." *Optometry* 80(12) (Dec 2009):695–701.

[215] Hamel, C. "Retinitis Pigmentosa." *Orphanet J Rare Dis* 1(2006):40. Hartong, D.T., E.L. Berson, T.P. Dryja. "Retinitis Pigmentosa." *Lancet* 368(9549) (Nov 18, 2006):1795–1809.

[216] Hamel, C. "Retinitis Pigmentosa." *Orphanet J Rare Dis* 1(2006):40. Berger, W., B. Kloeckener-Gruissem, J. Neidhardt. "The Molecular Basis of Human Retinal and Vitreoretinal Diseases." *Prog Retin Eye Res* 29(5) (Sep 29, 2010):335–375.

[217] Punzo, C., K. Kornacker, C.L. Cepko. "Stimulation of the Insulin/mTOR Pathway Delays Cone Death in a Mouse Model of Retinitis

Pigmentosa." *Nat Neurosci* 12(1) (Jan 2009):44–52.

[218] Koenekoop, R.K. "The Gene for Stargardt Disease, ABCA4, Is a Major Retinal Gene: A Mini-Review." *Ophthalmic Genet.* 24(2) (Jur 2003):75–80.

[219] Hartong, D.T., E.L. Berson, T.P. Dryja. "Retinitis Pigmentosa." *Lancet* 368(9549) (Nov 18, 2006):1795–1809.

[220] Tanito, M., S. Kaidzu, R.E. Anderson. "Delayed Loss of Cone and Remaining Rod Photoreceptor Cells Due to Impairment of Choroidal Circulation After Acute Light Exposure in Rats." *Invest Ophthalmol Vis Sci.* 48(4) (Apr 2007):1864–1872.

[221] Marc, R.E., B.W. Jones. "Retinal Remodeling in Inherited Photoreceptor Degenerations." *Mol Neurobiol 28(2)* (Oct 2003):139–147 Marc, R.E., B.W. Jones, C.B. Watt, et al. "Extreme Retinal Remodeling Triggered by Light Damage: Implications for Age Related Macular Degeneration." *Mol Vis* 14 (Apr 25, 2008):782–806.

[222] Punzo, C., K. Kornacker, C.L. Cepko. "Stimulation of the Insulin/mTOR Pathway Delays Cone Death in a Mouse Model of Retinitis Pigmentosa." *Nat Neurosci* 12(1) (Jan 2009):44–52.

[223] Komeima, K., B.S. Rogers, L. Lu, et al. "Antioxidants Reduce Cone Cell Death in a Model

of Retinitis Pigmentosa." *Proc Natl Acad Sci USA* 103(30) (Jul 25, 2006):11300–11305. Komeima, K., B.S. Rogers, P.A. Campochiaro. "Antioxidants Slow Photoreceptor Cell Death in Mouse Models of Retinitis Pigmentosa." *J Cell Physiol* 213(3) (Dec 2007):809–815. Usui, S., K. Komeima, S.Y. Lee, et al. "Increased Expression of Cata-lase and Superoxide Dismutase 2 Reduces Cone Cell Death in Retinitis Pigmentosa." *Mol Ther* 17(5) (May 2009):778786.

[224] Bill, A., G.O. Sperber. "Control of Retinal and Choroidal Blood Flow." *Eye (Lond)* 4(Pt. 2) (1990):319–325.

[225] Komeima, K., B.S. Rogers, P.A. Campochiaro. "Antioxidants Slow Photoreceptor Cell Death in Mouse Models of Retinitis Pigmentosa." *J Cell Physiol* 213(3) (Dec 2007):809–815.

[226] Yu, D.-Y., S.J. Cringle. "Retinal Degeneration and Local Oxygen Metabolism." *Exp Eye Res* 80(6) (Jun 2005):745–751.

[227] Léveillard, T., J.A. Sahel. "Rod-Derived Cone Viability Factor for Treating Blinding Diseases: From Clinic to Redox Signaling." *Sci Transl Med* 2(26) (Apr 7, 2010):26ps16.

[228] Punzo, C., K. Kornacker, C.L. Cepko. "Stimulation of the Insulin/mTOR Pathway Delays Cone Death in a Mouse Model of Retinitis Pigmentosa." *Nat Neurosci* 12(1) (Jan 2009):44–52.

[229] Massof, R.W., G.A. Fishman. "How Strong is the Evidence That Nutritional Supplements Slow the Progression of Retinitis Pigmentosa?" *Arch Ophthalmol* 128(4) (Apr 2010):493–495.

[230] Berson, E.L., B. Rosner, M.A. Sandberg, et al. "A Randomized Trial of Vitamin A and Vitamin E Supplementation for Retinitis Pigmentosa." *Arch Ophthalmol* 111(6) (Jun 1993):761–772.

[231] Mehta, J., D. Li, J.L. Mehta. "Vitamins C and E Prolong Time to Arterial Thrombosis in Rats." *J Nutr* 129(1) (Jan 1999):109–112.

[232] Head, K.A. "Natural Therapies for Ocular Disorders, Part One: Diseases of the Retina." *Altern Med Rev* 4(5) (Oct 1999):342–359.

[233] Yokota, T., T. Shiojiri, T. Gotoda, et al. "Retinitis Pigmentosa and Ataxia Caused by a Mutation in the Gene for the Alpha-Tocopherol Transfer Protein." *N Engl J Med* 335 (1996):1770–1771. Yokota, T., T. Uchihara, J. Kumagai, et al. "Postmortem Study of Ataxia with Retinitis Pigmentosa by Mutation of the?-Tocopherol-Transfer Protein Gene." *J Neurol Neurosurg Psychiatry* 68(4) (Apr 2000):521–525. Pang, J., M. Kiyosawa, Y. Seko, et al. "Clinicopathological Report of Retinitis Pigmentosa with Vitamin E Deficiency Caused by Mutation of the Alpha-Tocopherol Transfer Protein Gene." *Jpn J Ophthalmol* 45(6) (Nov-Dec 2001):672–676. Engin, K.N.

"Alpha-Tocopherol: Looking Beyond an Antioxidant." *Mol Vis* 15 (2009):855–860. Kono, S., A. Otsuji, H. Hattori, et al. "Ataxia with Vitamin E Deficiency with a Mutation in a Phospholipid Transfer Protein Gene." *J Neurol* 256(7) (Jul 2009):1180–1181.

[234] Yokota, T., T. Shiojiri, T. Gotoda, et al. "Retinitis Pigmentosa and Ataxia Caused by a Mutation in the Gene for the ?-Tocopherol-Transfer Protein." *N Engl J Med* 335 (1996):1770–1771.

[235] Head, K.A. "Natural Therapies for Ocular Disorders, Part One: Diseases of the Retina." *Altern Med Rev* 4(5) (Oct 1999):342–359.

[236] Organisciak, D.T., H.M. Wang, Z.Y. Li, et al. "The Protective Effect of Ascorbate in Retinal Light Damage of Rats." *Invest Ophthalmoi Vis Sci* 26(11) (Nov 1985):1580–1588. Hamel, C. "Retinitis Pigmentosa." *Orphanet J Rare Dis* 1(2006):40. Komeima, K., B.S. Rogers, L. Lu, el al. "Antioxidants Reduce Cone Cell Death in a Model of Retinitis Pigmentosa." *Proc Natl Acad Sci* USA 103(30) (Jul 25, 2006):11300–11305.

[237] Mathews, L., K. Narayanadas, G. Sunil. "Thiamine Responsive Megaloblastic Anemia." *Indian Pediatr 46(2)* (Feb 2009):172–174.

[238] Komeima, K., B.S. Rogers, L. Lu, et al. "Antioxidants Reduce Cone Cell Death in a Model of Retinitis Pigmentosa." *Proc Natl Acad Sci*

USA 103(30) (Jul 25, 2006):11300–11305. Komeima, K., B.S. Rogers, P.A. Campochiaro. "Antioxidants Slow Photoreceptor Cell Death in Mouse Models of Retinitis Pigmentosa." *J Cell Physiol* 213(3) (Dec 2007):809–815.

[239] Ma, L., X.M. Lin. "Effects of Lutein and Zeaxanthin on Aspects of Eye Health." *J Sci Food Agric* 90(1) (Jan 2010):2–12.

[240] Neustadt, J., S.R. Pieczenik. "Medication-Induced Mitochondrial Damage and Disease." *Mol Nutr Food Res* 52(7) (Jul 2008):780–788.

[241] Massof, R.W., D. Finkelstein. "Supplemental Vitamin A Retards Loss of ERG Amplitude in Retinitis Pigmentosa." *Arch Ophthalmo* 111 (6) (Jun 1993):751–754. Berson, E.L., B. Rosner, M.A. Sandberg, et al. "A Randomized Trial of Vitamin A and Vitamin E Supplementation for Retinitis Pigmentosa." *Arch Ophthalmol* 111(6) (Jun 1993):761–772. Berson, E.L., B. Rosner, M.A. Sandberg, et al "Clinical trial of docosahexaenoic acid in patients with retinitis pigmentosa receiving vitamin A treatment." *Arch Ophthalmol.* 122(9) (Sei 2004):1297–1305. Berson, E.L., B. Rosner, M.A. Sandberg, et al. "Further Evaluation of Docosahexaenoic Acid in Patients with Retiniti5 Pigmentosa Receiving Vitamin A Treatment: Subgroup Analyses." *Arch Ophthalmol* 122(9) (Sep 2004):1306–1314. Hamel, C. "Retiniti! Pigmentosa." *Orphanet J Rare Dis*

1(2006):40. Berson, E.L. "Long-Term Visual Prognoses in Patients with Retinitis Pigmentosa: The Ludwig von Sallmann Lecture." *Exp Eye Res* 85(1) (Jul 2007):7–14.

[242] Berson, E.L., B. Rosner, M.A. Sandberg, et al. "Clinical Trial of Lutein in Patients with Retinitis Pigmentosa Receiving Vitamin A." *Arch Ophthalmol* 128(4) (Apr 2010):403–411.

[243] Berson, E.L., B. Rosner, M.A. Sandberg, et al. "Further Evaluation of Docosa-hexaenoic Acid in Patients with Retinitis Pigmentosa Receiving Vitamin A Treatment: Subgroup Analyses." *Arch Ophthalmol* 122(9) (Sep 2004):1306–1314.

[244] Hartong, D.T., E.L. Berson, T.P. Dryja. "Retinitis pigmentosa." *Lancet* 368(9549) (Nov 18, 2006):1795–1809.

[245] Fine, L.C., J.S. Heier. *The Aging Eye: Preventing and Treating Eye Disease.* Special Health Reports. Boston, MA: Harvard Medical School, 2010.

Chapter 6. Vitamins Prevent Degeneration of Retinal Ganglion Cells: Glaucoma, Diabetic Retinopathy

[246] Harris, A., C. Jonescu-Cuypers, B. Martin, et al. "Simultaneous Management of Blood Flow and IOP in Glaucoma." *Acta Ophthalmo Scand* 79(4) (Aug 2001):336–341.

[247] Tezel, G.. "Oxidative Stress in Glaucomatous Neurodegeneration: Mechanisms and Consequences." *Prog Retin Eye Res* 25(5) (Sep 2006):490–513. Mozaffarieh, M., J. Flammer. "A Novel Perspective on Natural Therapeutic Approaches in Glaucoma Therapy." *Expert Opin Emerging Drugs* 12(2) (May 2007):195–198.

[248] Oshida, E., Y. Matsumoto, K. Arai. "Free Radicals in the Aqueous Humor of Patients with Glaucoma." *Clin Ophthalmol* 4 (Jul 30, 2010):653–660.

[249] Yuki, K., D. Murat, I. Kimura, et al. "Reduced-Serum Vitamin C and Increased Uric Acid Levels in Normal-Tension Glaucoma." *Graefes Arch Clin Exp Ophthalmol* 248(2) (Feb 2010):243–248.

[250] Izzotti, A., A. Bagnis, S.C. Saccàa. "The Role of Oxidative Stress in Glaucoma." *Mutat Res* 612(2) (Mar 2006):105–114. Schober, M.S., G. Chidlow, J.P. Wood, et al. "Bioenergetic-Based Neuroprotection and Glaucoma." *Clin Experiment Ophthalmol* 36(4) (May 2008):377–385.

[251] Osborne, N.N. "Pathogenesis of Ganglion "Cell Death" in Glaucoma and Neuroprotection: Focus on Ganglion Cell Axonal Mitochondria." *Prog Brain Res* 173 (2008):339–352.

[252] Balaratnasingam, C., W.H. Morgan, L. Bass, et al. "Time-Dependent Effects of Focal Retinal

Ischemia on Axonal Cytoskeleton Proteins." *Invest Ophthalmol Vis Sci.* 51(6) (Jun 2010):3019–3028.

[253] Osborne, N.N. "Pathogenesis of Ganglion "Cell Death" in Glaucoma and Neuroprotection: Focus on Ganglion Cell Axonal Mitochondria." *Prog Brain Res* 173 (2008):339–352.

[254] Arnarsson. A.M. "Epidemiology of Exfoliation Syndrome in the Reykjavik Eye Study." *Acta Ophthalmol* 87 (Dec 2009)Thesis 3:1–17.

[255] Izzotti, A., A. Bagnis, S.C. Saccà. "The Role of Oxidative Stress in Glaucoma." *Mutat Res* 612(2) (Mar 2006):105–114. Saccà, S.C., A Izzotti. "Oxidative Stress and Glaucoma: Injury in the Anterior Segment of the Eye." *Prog Brain Res* 173 (2008):385–407. Izzotti, A., S. C Sacca, M. Longobardi, et al. "Mitochondrial Damage in the Trabecular Meshwork of Patients with Glaucoma." *Arch Ophthalmol* 128(6) (Jun 2010):724–730.

[256] Dean, C. *The Magnesium Miracle.* New York, NY: Ballantine, 2007.

[257] Mozaffarieh, M., J. Flammer. "A Novel Perspective on Natural Therapeutic Approaches in Glaucoma Therapy." *Expert Opin Emerging Drugs* 12(2) (May 2007):195–198.

[258] Linnér, E. "The Pressure Lowering Effect of Ascorbic Acid in Ocular Hypertension." *Acta Ophthalmol (Copenh)* 47(3) (1969):685–689 Boyd, H.H. "Eye Pressure Lowering Effect of

Vitamin *C.*" *J Orthomol Med* 10 (1995):165–168.

[259] Head, K.A. "Natural Therapies for Ocular Disorders, Part Two: Cataracts and Glaucoma." *Altern Med Rev* 6(2) (Apr 2001):141–166.

[260] Linnér, E. "The Pressure Lowering Effect of Ascorbic Acid in Ocular Hypertension." *Acta Ophthalmol (Copenh)* 47(3) (1969):685–689 Boyd, H.H. "Eye Pressure Lowering Effect of Vitamin C." *J Orthomol Med* 10 (1995):165–168. Head, K.A. "Natural Therapies for Ocular Disorders, Part Two: Cataracts and Glaucoma." *Altern Med Rev* 6(2) (Apr 2001):141–166.

[261] Schober, M.S., G. Chidlow, J.P. Wood, et al. "Bioenergetic-Based Neuroprotection and Glaucoma." *Clin Experiment Ophthalmol* 36(4) (May 2008):377–385.

[262] Coleman, A.L., K.L. Stone, G. Kodjebacheva et al. "Glaucoma Risk and the Consumption of Fruits and Vegetables Among Oldei Women in the Study of Osteoporotic Fractures." *Am J Ophthalmol* 145(6) (Jun 2008):1081–1089.

[263] United States Department of Agriculture. "SR23 Page Reports." List of Nutrient Content in Foods, http://www.ars.usda.gov/Services/docs.htm?docid=20957. United States Department of Agriculture. "SR23 Reports by Single Nutrients" http://www.ars.usda.gov/Services

/docs.htm?docid=20958. (accessed Aug 2011).

[264] Coleman, A.L., K.L. Stone, G. Kodjebacheva et al. "Glaucoma Risk and the Consumption of Fruits and Vegetables Among Oldei Women in the Study of Osteoporotic Fractures." *Am J Ophthalmol* 145(6) (Jun 2008):1081–1089.

[265] Ferreira, S.M., S.F. Lerner, R. Brunzini, et al. "Antioxidant Status in the Aqueous Humour of Patients with Glaucoma Associated with Exfoliation Syndrome." *Eye (Lond)* 23(8) (Aug 2009):1691–1697.

[266] Osborne, N.N. "Pathogenesis of Ganglion "Cell Death" in Glaucoma and Neuroprotection: Focus on Ganglion Cell Axona Mitochondria." *Prog Brain Res* 173 (2008):339–352.

[267] Veach, J. "Functional Dichotomy: Glutathione and Vitamin E in Homeostasis Relevant to Primary Open-Angle Glaucoma." *Br J Nut* 91(6) (Jun 2004):809–829.

[268] Engin, K.N. "Alpha-Tocopherol: Looking Beyond an Antioxidant." *Mol Vis* 15 (2009):855–860.

[269] Ko, M.L., P.H. Peng, S.Y. Hsu, et al. "Dietary Deficiency of Vitamin E Aggravates Retinal Ganglion Cell Death in Experimental Glaucoma of Rats." *Curr Eye Res* 35(9) (Sep 2010):842–849.

[270] Bartlett, H.E., F. Eperjesi. "Nutritional Supplementation for Type 2 Diabetes: A System-

atic Review." *Ophthalmic Physiol Opt 28(6)* (Nov 2008):503–523.

[271] Head, K.A. "Natural Therapies for Ocular Disorders, Part One: Diseases of the Retina." *Altern Med Rev 4(5)* (Oct 1999):342–359.

[272] Maritim, A.C., R.A. Sanders, J.B. Watkins, III. "Diabetes, Oxidative Stress, and Antioxidants: A Review." *J Biochem Mol Toxicol* 17(1) (2003):24–38.

[273] Chrissobolis, S., A.A. Miller, G.R. Drummond, et al. "Oxidative Stress and Endothelial Dysfunction in Cerebrovascular Disease." *Front Biosci* 16 (Jan 1, 2011):1733–1745.

[274] Ciudin, A., C. Hernandez, R. Simo. "Iron Overload in Diabetic Retinopathy: A Cause or a Consequence of Impaired Mechanisms?" *Exp Diabetes Res* 2010 (2010):pli 714–108.

[275] Bartlett, H.E., F. Eperjesi. "Nutritional Supplementation for Type 2 Diabetes: A Systematic Review." *Ophthalmic Physiol Opt 28(6)* (Nov 2008):503–523.

[276] Harding, A.H., N.J. Wareham, S.A. Bingham, et al. "Plasma Vitamin C Level, Fruit and Vegetable Consumption, and the Risk of New On set Type 2 Diabetes Mellitus: The European Prospective Investigation of Cancer-Norfolk Prospective Study." *Arch Intern Med* 168(14) (Jul 28, 2008):1493–1499.

[277] Frikke-Schmidt, H., P. Tveden-Nyborg, M.M. Birck, et al. "High Dietary Fat and Cholesterol

Exacerbates Chronic Vitamin C Deficiency in Guinea Pigs." *Br J Nutr* 105(1) (Jan 2011):54–61.

[278] Shargorodsky, M., O. Debby, Z. Matas, et al. "Effect of Long-Term Treatment with Antioxidants (Vitamin C, Vitamin E, Coenzyme Q_{10} and Selenium) on Arterial Compliance, Humoral Factors and Inflammatory Markers in Patients with Multiple Cardiovascular Risk Factors." *Nutr Metab (Lond)* 7 (Jul 6,2010):55.

[279] Bartlett, H.E., F. Eperjesi. "Nutritional Supplementation for Type 2 Diabetes: A Systematic Review." *Ophthalmic Physiol Opt* 28(6) (Nov 2008):503–523.

[280] Bursell, S.E., A.C. Clermont, L.P. Aiello et al. "High-Dose Vitamin E Supplementation Normalizes Retinal Blood Flow and Creatinine Clearance in Patients with Type 1 Diabetes." *Diabetes Care* 22(8) (Aug 1999):1245–1251. Bartlett, H.E., F. Eperjesi. "Nutritional Supplementation for Type 2 Diabetes: A Systematic Review." *Ophthalmic Physiol Opt* 28(6) (Nov 2008):503–523. Pazdro, R., J.R. Burgess "The Role of Vitamin E and Oxidative Stress in Diabetes Complications." *Mech Ageing Dev* 131(4) (Apr 2010):276–286.

[281] Boyd, H.H. "Eye Pressure Lowering Effect of Vitamin *C." J Orthomol Med* 10 (1995):165–168.

[282] Witham, M.D., F.J. Dove, M. Dryburgh, et al. "The Effect of Different Doses of Vitamin D(3) on Markers of Vascular Health in Patients with Type 2 Diabetes: A Randomised Controlled Trial." *Diabetologia* 53(10) (Oct 2010):2112–2119.

[283] McNair, P., C. Christiansen, S. Madsbad, et al. "Hypomagnesemia, a Risk Factor in Diabetic Retinopathy." *Diabetes* 27(11) (NoN 1978):1075–1077. Mather, H.M., J.A. Nisbet, G.H. Burton, et al. "Hypomagnesaemia in Diabetes." *Clin Chim Acta* 95(2) (Jul 16, 1979):235242. Walter, Jr, R.M., J.Y. Uriu-Hare, K.L. Olin, et al. "Copper, Zinc, Manganese, and Magnesium Status and Complications of Diabetes Mellitus." *Diabetes Care* 14(11) (Nov 1991):1050–1056.

[284] Dean, C. *The Magnesium Miracle.* New York, NY: Ballantine, 2007.

[285] Harding, A.H., N.J. Wareham, S.A. Bingham, et al. "Plasma Vitamin C Level, Fruit and Vegetable Consumption, and the Risk of New On set Type 2 Diabetes Mellitus: The European Prospective Investigation of Cancer-Norfolk Prospective Study." *Arch Intern Med* 168(14) (Jul 28, 2008):1493–1499. Trapp, C.B., N.D. Barnard. "Usefulness of Vegetarian and Vegan diets for Treating Type 2 Diabetes." *Curr Dial Rep* 10(2) (Apr 2010):152–158.

[286] Becker, G.. *The First Year. Type 2 Diabetes: An Essential Guide for the Newly Diagnosed.* 2nd ed., Cambridge, MA: Da Capo Press, 2006 Barnard, N.D. *Dr. Neal Barnard's Program for Reversing Diabetes: The Scientifically Proven System for Reversing Diabetes without Drugs.* New York, NY: Rodale Books, 2008. Magee, E. *Tell Me What to Eat If I Have Diabetes: Nutrition You Can Live With.* Rev., 3rd ed., Franklir Lakes, NJ: New Page Books, 2009.

Chapter 7. Vitamins for Other Conditions and Diseases of the Eye

[287] Kim, E.C., J.S. Choi, C.K. Joo. "A Comparison of Vitamin A and Cyclosporine A 0.05% Eye Drops for Treatment of Dry Eye Syndrome." *Am J Ophthalmol* 147(2) (Feb 2009):206–213.

[288] Ibid.

[289] Gaby, A.R. "Nutritional Therapies for Ocular Disorders: Part Three." *Altern Med Rev* 13(3) (Sep 2008):191–204.

[290] Ibid.

[291] Maggini, S., E.S. Wintergerst, S. Beveridge, et al. "Selected Vitamins and Trace Elements Support Immune Function by Strengthening Epithelial Barriers and Cellular and Humoral Immune Responses." *Br J Nutr* 98 Suppl 1 (Oct 2007):S29–35.

[292] Gaby, A.R. "Nutritional Therapies for Ocular Disorders: Part Three." *Altern Med Rev* 13(3) (Sep 2008):191–204.

[293] Raczynska, K., B. Iwaszkiewicz-Bilikiewicz, W. Stozkowska, et al. "Clinical Evaluation of Provitamin B_5 Drops and Gel for Postoperative Treatment of Corneal and Conjuctival Injuries." *Klin Oczna* 105(3-4) (2003):175–178. Gaby, A.R. "Nutritional Therapies for Ocular Disorders: Part Three." *Altern Med Rev* 13(3) (Sep 2008):191–204.

[294] Yadav, U.C., N.M. Kalariya, K.V. Ramana. "Emerging Role of Antioxidants in the Protection of Uveitis Complications." *Curr Med Chem* 18(6) (2011):931–42.

[295] Keino, H., T. Watanabe, Y. Sato, et al. "Anti-Inflammatory Effect of Retinoic Acid on Experimental Auto immune Uveoretinitis." *Br J Ophthalmol* 94(6) (Jun 2010):802–807.

[296] Saul, *A. Doctor Yourself. Natural Healing That Works.* Laguna Beach, CA: Basic Health Publications, 2003.

[297] Gaby, A.R. "Nutritional Therapies for Ocular Disorders: Part Three." *Altern Med Rev* 13(3) (Sep 2008):191–204.

[298] Makdoumi, K., I. Mortensen, S. Crafoord. "Infectious Keratitis Treated with Corneal Crosslinking." *Cornea* 29(12) (Dec 2010):13531358.

[299] Mencucci, R., M. Marini, I. Paladini, et al. “Effects of Riboflavin/UVA Corneal Cross-Linking on Keratocytes and Collagen Fibres in Human Cornea.” *Clin Experiment Ophthalmol.* 38(1) (Jan 2010):49–56.

[300] Vinciguerra, P., F.I. Camesasca, D. Ponzin. “Use of Amino Acids in Refractive Surgery.” *J Refract Surg* 18(3 Suppl) (May-Jun 2002):5374–377.

[301] Wishard, P., C.A. Paterson. “The Effect of Ascorbic Acid on Experimental Acid Burns of the Rabbit Cornea.” *Invest Ophthalmol Vis Sci* 19(5) (May 1980):564–566. Pfister, R.R., J.L. Haddox, D. Yuille-Barr. “The Combined Effect of Citrate/Ascorbate Treatment in Alkali-Injured Rabbit Eyes.” *Cornea* 10(2) (Mar 1991):100–104.

[302] Chan, D., S.R. Lamande, W.G. Cole, et al. “Regulation of Procollagen Synthesis and Processing During Ascorbate-Induced Extracellular Matrix Accumulation in Vitro” *Biochem J* 269(1) (Jul 1, 1990):175–181. Phu, D., E.J. Orwin. “Characterizing the Effects o] Aligned Collagen Fibers and Ascorbic Acid Derivatives on Behavior of Rabbit Corneal Fibroblasts.” *Conf Proc IEEE Eng Med Biol Soc* 2005 (2009):4242–4245.

[303] Serbecic, N., S.C. Beutelspacher. “Anti-Oxidative Vitamins Prevent Lipid-Peroxidation and

Apoptosis in Corneal Endothelial Cells." *Cell Tissue Res* 320(3) (Jun 2005):465–475.

[304] Berthout, A., M. Sellam, F. Denimal, et al. "The Eye and Anorexia Nervosa. A Case Report." *J Fr Ophtalmol* 30(6) (Jun 2007):e15.

[305] Opstelten, W., J. Eekhof, A.K. Neven, et al. "Treatment of Herpes Zoster." *Can Fam Physician* 54(3) (Mar 2008):373–377.

[306] Levy, T.E. *Curing the Incurable: Vitamin C, Infectious Diseases, and Toxins.* Henderson, NV: LivOn Books, 2002.

[307] Maggini, S., E.S. Wintergerst, S. Beveridge, et al. "Selected Vitamins and Trace Elements Support Immune Function by Strengthening Epithelial Barriers and Cellular and Humoral Immune Responses." *Br J Nutr* 98 Suppl 1 (Oct 2007):529–35.

[308] Pacholok, S.M., J.J. Stuart. *Could It Be B_{12}: An Epidemic of Misdiagnoses.* Sanger, CA: Quill Driver Books/Word Dancer Press, 2005.

[309] Johnson, M.W. "Perifoveal Vitreous Detachment and Its Macular Complications." *Trans Am Ophthalmol Soc* 103 (Dec 2005):537–567.

[310] Johnson, M.W. "Perifoveal Vitreous Detachment and Its Macular Complications." *Trans Am Ophthalmol Soc* 103 (Dec 2005):537–567. Sendrowski, D.P., M.A. Bronstein. "Current Treatment for Vitreous Floaters." *Optometry* 81(3) (Mar 2010):157–161.

[311] Johnson, M.W. "Perifoveal Vitreous Detachment and Its Macular Complications." *Trans Am Ophthalmol Soc* 103 (Dec 2005):537–567.

[312] Ibid.

[313] Ibid.

[314] Chen, W.Y. J., G. Abatangelo. "Functions of Hyaluronan in Wound Repair." *Wound Repair Regen* 7(2) (Mar-Apr 1999):79–89.

[315] Graves, J., L.J. Balcer. "Eye Disorders in Patients with Multiple Sclerosis: Natural History and Management." *Clin Ophthalmol* (2010):1409–1422.

[316] Garcia-Martin, E., V. Pueyo, J. Ara, et al. "Effect of Optic Neuritis on Progressive Axonal Damage in Multiple Sclerosis Patients." *Mul Scler J* 17(7) (Jul 2011)830-837.

[317] Graves, J., L.J. Balcer. "Eye Disorders in Patients with Multiple Sclerosis: Natural History and Management." *Clin Ophthalmol 4* (2010):1409–1422. Matti, S., F. Lolli. "Neuromyelitis Optica: An Update." *J Neurol Sci* 303(1-2) (Apr 2011):13–21

[318] Simpson, S. Jr., B. Taylor, L. Blizzard, et al. "Higher 25-Hydroxyvitamin D is Associated with Lower Relapse Riskin Multiple Sclerosis." *Ann Neurol* 68(2) (Aug 2010):193–203.

Lucas, R.M., A.L. Ponsonby, K. Dear, et al. "Sun Exposure and Vitamin D Are Independent

Risk Factors for CNS Demyelination." *Neurology* 76(6) (Feb 8 2011):540–548.

[319] Levy, T.E. *Curing the Incurable: Vitamin C, Infectious Diseases, and Toxins.* Henderson, NV: LivOn Books, 2002.

[320] Levy, T.E. *Stop America's #1 Killer: Reversible Vitamin Deficiency Found to be Origin of All Coronary Heart Disease.* Henderson, NV: LivOn Books, 2006.

[321] Kurl, S., T.P. Tuomainen, J.A. Laukkanen, et al. "Plasma Vitamin C Modifies the Association between Hypertension and Risk of Stroke." *Stroke* 33(6) (Jun 2002):1568–1573. Levy, T.E. *Stop America's #1 Killer: Reversible Vitamin Deficiency Found to be Origin of All Coronary Heart Disease.* Henderson, NV: LivOn Books, 2006.

[322] Schiirks, M., R.J. Glynn, P.M. Rist, et al. "Effects of Vitamin E on Stroke Subtypes: Meta-Analysis of Randomised Controlled Trials." *BMJ.* 341 (Nov 4, 2010):c5702.

[323] Collier, B.R., A. Giladi, L.A. Dossett, et al. "Impact of High-Dose Antioxidants on Outcomes in Acutely Injured Patients." *JPEN J Parenter Enteral Nutr* 32(4) (Jul-Aug 2008):384–388.

[324] Kahn, S.A., R.J. Beers, C.W. Lentz. "Resuscitation after Severe Burn Injury Using High-Dose Ascorbic Acid: A Retrospective Review."

J Burn Care Res 32(1) (Jan-Feb 2011):110–117.

[325] Nathens, A.B., M.J. Neff, G.J. Jurkovich, et al. "Randomized, Prospective Trial of Antioxidant Supplementation in Critically Ill Surgical Patients." *Ann Surg* 236(6) (Dec 2002):814–822.

[326] Weitzel, L.R., W.J. Mayles, P.A. Sandoval, et al. "Effects of Pharmaconutrients on Cellular Dysfunction and the Micro circulation in Critical Illness." *Curr Opin Anaesthesiol* 22(2) (Apr 2009):177–183.

[327] Gross, R.L. "Collagen Type I and III Synthesis by Tenon's Capsule Fibroblasts in Culture: Individual Patient Characteristics and Response to Mitomycin C, 5-Fluorouracil, and Ascorbic Acid." *Trans Am Ophthalmol Soc* 97 (1999):513–543. Leite, M.T., T.S. Prata, C.Z. Kera, et al. "Ascorbic Acid Concentration is Reduced in the Secondary Aqueous Humour of Glaucomatous Patients." *Clin Experiment Ophthalmol* 37(4) (May 2009):402–406.

[328] Reiss, G.. R., P.G. Werness, P.E. Zollman, et al. "Ascorbic Acid Levels in the Aqueous Humor of Nocturnal and Diurnal Mammals." *Arch Ophthalmol* 104(5) (May 1986):753–755.

[329] Gross, R.L. "The Effect of Ascorbate on Wound Healing." *Int Ophthalmol Clin.* 40(4) (Fall 2000):51–57.

[330] Hoffer, A., A.W. Saul. *Orthomolecular Medicine for Everyone: Megavitamin Therapeutics for Families and Physicians.* Laguna Beach CA: Basic Health Publications, 2008.

[331] Vinciguerra, P., F.I. Camesasca, D. Ponzin. "Use of Amino Acids in Refractive Surgery." *J Refract Surg* 18(3 Suppl) (May-Jur 2002):5374–377.

[332] Urgancioglu, B., K. Bilgihan, D. Engin, et al. "Topical N-Acetylcysteine Reduces Interleukin-1-Alpha in Tear Fluid After Laser Subepithelial Keratectomy." *Eur J Ophthalmol* 19(4) (Jul-Aug 2009):554–559.

[333] Perrone, S., S. Negro, M.L. Tataranno, et al. "Oxidative Stress and Antioxidant Strategies in Newborns." *J Matern Fetal Neonatal Mec* 23(Suppl 3) (Oct 2010):63–5.

[334] Lien, E.L., B.R. Hammond. "Nutritional Influences on Visual Development and Function." *Prog Retin Eye Res* 30(3) (May 2011):188203.

[335] Lee, J.W., J.M. Davis. "Future Applications of Antioxidants in Premature Infants." *Curr Opin Pediatr* 23(2) (Apr 2011):161–166.

[336] Cringle, S.J., D.Y. Yu. "Oxygen Supply and Consumption in the Retina: Implications for Studies of Retinopathy of Prematurity." *Doc Ophthalmol* 120(1) (Feb 2010):99–109.

[337] Lien, E.L., B.R. Hammond. "Nutritional Influences on Visual Development and Function."

Prog Retin Eye Res 30(3) (May 2011):188203.
[338] Lee, J.W., J.M. Davis. "Future Applications of Antioxidants in Premature Infants." *Curr Opin Pediatr* 23(2) (Apr 2011):161–166.
[339] Emery, T.F. *Iron and your Health: Facts and Fallacies.* Boca Raton, FL: CRC Press, 1991.
[340] Lien, E.L., B.R. Hammond. "Nutritional Influences on Visual Development and Function." *Prog Retin Eye Res* 30(3) (May 2011):188203.
[341] Ibid.
[342] Ibid.
[343] Ibid.

Chapter 8. Eating Right to Prevent Eye Disease

[344] Head, K.A. "Natural Therapies for Ocular Disorders, Part One: Diseases of the Retina." *Altern Med Rev* 4(5) (Oct 1999):342–359. Head, K.A. "Natural Therapies for Ocular Disorders, Part Two: Cataracts and Glaucoma." *Altern Med Rev* 6(2) (Apr 2001):141–166. Gaby, A.R. "Nutritional Therapies for Ocular Disorders: Part Three." *Altern Med Rev* 13(3) (Sep 2008):191–204.
[345] Elsas, L.J., P.B. Acosta. "Nutritional Support of Inherited Metabolic Diseases." Chapter 61 in *Modern Nutrition in Health and Disease,*

editors M.E. Shils, J.A. Olson, M. Shike, et al., 9th ed. Baltimore, MD: Williams & Wilkins, 1999.

[346] Pauling, L. *How to Live Longer And Feel Better.* Corvallis, OR: Oregon State University Press, 1986, 2006. Hoffer, A., A.W. Saul. *Orthomolecular Medicine for Everyone: Megavitamin Therapeutics for Families and Physicians.* Laguna Beach, CA: Basic Health Publications, 2008.

[347] Pauling, L. *How to Live Longer And Feel Better.* Corvallis, OR: Oregon State University Press, 1986, 2006.

[348] Carper, J. *Food: Your Miracle Medicine.* New York, NY: HarperCollins, 1998. Levy, T.E. *Optimal Nutrition for Optimal Health.* Chicago, IL: Keats Publishing, 2001. Saul, A. *Doctor Yourself: Natural Healing That Works.* Laguna Beach, CA: Basic Health Publications, 2003. McGee, H. *On Food and Cooking: The Science and Lore of the Kitchen.* New York, NY: Scribner, Revised, updated edition, 2004. United States Department of Agriculture. "SR23 Page Reports." List of Nutrient Content in Foods. http://www.ars.usda.gov/Services/docs.htm?docid=20957. United States Department of Agriculture. "SR23 Reports by Single Nutrients." http://www.ars.usda.gov/Services/docs.htm?docid=20958 . (accessed Aug 2011).

[349] Levy, T. E. *Optimal Nutrition for Optimal Health.* Chicago, IL: Keats Publishing, 2001.

[350] Saul, A. *Doctor Yourself: Natural Healing That Works.* Laguna Beach, CA: Basic Health Publications, 2003.

[351] Boutenko, V. *Green for Life.* Berkely, CA: North Atlantic Books, 2010.

[352] United States Department of Agriculture. "SR23Page Reports." List of Nutrient Content in Foods. http://www.ars.usda.gov/Services/docs.htm?docid=20957 .

[353] Coleman, A.L., K.L. Stone, G. Kodjebacheva et al. "Glaucoma Risk and the Consumption of Fruits and Vegetables Among Older Women in the Study of Osteoporotic Fractures." *Am J Ophthalmol* 145(6) (Jun 2008):1081–1089.

[354] United States Department of Agriculture. "SR23 Page Reports." List of Nutrient Content in Foods. http://www.ars.usda.gov/Services/docs.htm?docid=20957 . (accessed Aug 2011).

[355] Sesso, H.D., J.E. Buring, W.G. Christen, et al. "Vitamins E and C in the Prevention of Cardiovascular Disease in Men: The Physicians' Health Study II Randomized Controlled Trial." *JAMA* 300(18) (Nov 12, 2008):2123–2133.

[356] Fletcher, A.E. "Controversy over "Contradiction": Should Randomized Trials Always Trump

Observational Studies?" *Am J Ophthalmol* 147(3) (Mar 2009):384–386.

[357] Ibid.

[358] Ibid.

[359] Houston, M.C. "The Role of Cellular Micronutrient Analysis, Nutraceuticals, Vitamins, Antioxidants and Minerals in the Prevention and Treatment of Hypertension and Cardiovascular Disease." *Ther Adv Cardiovasc Dis* 4(3) (Jun 2010):165–183.

[360] Millen, A.E., M. Gruber, R. Klein, et al. "Relations of Serum Ascorbic Acid and Alpha-Tocopherol to Diabetic Retinopathy in the Third National Health and Nutrition Examination Survey." *Am J Epidemiol* 158(3) (Aug 1, 2003):225–233.

[361] Fine, L.C., J.S. Heier. *The Aging Eye: Preventing and Treating Eye Disease.* Special Health Reports. Boston, MA: Harvard Medical School, 2010.

[362] International Agency for Research on Cancer. *IARC Monographs on the Evaluation of Carcinogenic Risks to Humans: Tobacco Smoke and Involuntary Smoking.* Volume 83 (2004). Available from http://www.iarc.fr.

[363] Bertram, K.M., C.J. Baglole, R.P. Phipps, et al. "Molecular Regulation of Cigarette Smoke Induced-Oxidative Stress in Human Retinal Pigment Epithelial Cells: Implications for Age-

Related Macular Degeneration." *Am J Physiol Cell Physiol* 297(5) (Nov 2009):C1200–1210.

[364] Hiller, R., R.D. Sperduto, M.J. Podgor, et al. "Cigarette Smoking and the Risk of Development of Lens Opacities. The Framingham Studies." *Arch Ophthalmol* 115(9) (Sep 1997):1113–1118. Mares, J.A., R. Voland, R. Adler R, et al.; CAREDS Group. "Healthy Diets and the Subsequent Prevalence of Nuclear Cataract in Women." *Arch Ophthalmol* 128(6) (Jun 2010):738–749.

[365] Handelman, G.J., L. Packer, C.E. Cross. "Destruction of Tocopherols, Carotenoids, and Retinol in Human Plasma by Cigarette Smoke." *Am J Clin Nutr* 63 (1996):559–565. Frikke-Schmidt, H., P. Tveden-Nyborg, M.M. Birck, et al. "High Dietary Fat and Cholesterol Exacerbates Chronic Vitamin C Deficiency in Guinea Pigs." *Br J Nutr* 105(1) (Jan 2011):54–61.

[366] Mosad, S.M., A.A. Ghanem, H.M. El-Fallal, et al. "Lens Cadmium, Lead, and Serum Vitamins C, E, and Beta Carotene in Cataractous Smoking Patients." *Curr Eye Res* 35(1) (Jan 2010):23–30.

[367] Levy, T.E. *Curing the Incurable: Vitamin C, Infectious Diseases, and Toxins.* Henderson, NV: LivOn Books, 2002.

[368] de Jong, P.T. "Age-Related Macular Degeneration." *N Engl J Med* 355(14) (Oct 5,

2006):1474–1485. Bertram, K.M., C.J. Baglole, R.P. Phipps, et al. "Molecular Regulation of Cigarette Smoke Induced-Oxidative Stress in Human Retinal Pigment Epithelial Cells: Implications for Age-Related Macular Degeneration." *Am J Physiol Cell Physiol* 297(5) (Nov 2009):C1200–1210.

[369] Evans, J.R., A.E. Fletcher, R.P. Wormald. "28,000 Cases of Age Related Macular Degeneration Causing Visual Loss in People Aged 75 Years and Above in the United Kingdom May Be Attributable to Smoking." *Br J Ophthalmol* 89(5) (May 2005):550–553. de Jong, P.T. "Age-Related Macular Degeneration. *N Engl J Med* 355(14) (Oct 5, 2006):1474–1485.

[370] Tan, J.S., J.J. Wang, V. Flood, et al. "Dietary Antioxidants and the Long-Term Incidence of Age-Related Macular Degeneration: The Blue Mountains Eye Study." *Ophthalmology* 115(2) (Feb 2008):334–341.

[371] Bertram, K.M., C.J. Baglole, R.P. Phipps, et al. "Molecular Regulation of Cigarette Smoke Induced-Oxidative Stress in Human Retinal Pigment Epithelial Cells: Implications for Age-Related Macular Degeneration." *Am J Physiol Cell Physiol* 297(5) (Nov 2009):C1200–1210.

[372] Ibid.

[373] Goralczyk, R. "Beta-Carotene and Lung Cancer in Smokers: Review of Hypotheses and

Status of Research." *Nutr Cancer* 61(6) (2009):767–774.

[374] Hemila, H., J. Kaprio. "Subgroup Analysis of Large Trials Can Guide Further Research: A Case Study of Vitamin E and Pneumonia." *Clin Epidemiol* 3 (2011):51–59.

[375] Hemila, H., J. Kaprio. "Vitamin E May Affect the Life Expectancy of Men, Depending on Dietary Vitamin C Intake and Smoking." *Age Ageing* 40(2) (Mar 2011):215–220.

[376] Ebbing, M., K.H. Bonaa, O. Nygard, et al. "Cancer Incidence and Mortality after Treatment With Folic Acid and Vitamin B_{12}." *JAMA* 302(19) (Nov 18, 2009):2119–2126.

[377] Ross, C.A. "Vitamin A and Retinoids." Chapter 17 in *Modern Nutrition in Health and Disease,* editors M.E. Shils, J.A. Olson, M. Shike et al., 9th ed. Baltimore, MD: Williams & Wilkins, 1999.

[378] Ibid.

[379] Ibid.

[380] Ross, C.A. "Vitamin A and Retinoids." Chapter 17 in *Modern Nutrition in Health and Disease,* editors M.E. Shils, J.A. Olson, M. Shike et al., 9th ed. Baltimore, MD: Williams & Wilkins, 1999. United States Department of Agriculture. Institute of Medicine (IOM), Food and Nutrition Information Center. National Academy of Sciences. "Dietary Reference Intakes for Vitamin A, Vitamin K, Arsenic, Boron,

Chromium, Copper, Iodine, Iron, Manganese, Molybdenum, Nickel, Silicon, Vanadium, and Zinc" (2001) Online at: http://fnic.nal.usda.gov/nal_display/index.php?info_center=4&tax_level=4&tax_subject=256&topic_id=1342&level3_id=5141&level4_id=10590. (accessed Aug 2011).

[381] Linseisen, J., S. Rohrmann, A.B. Miller, et al. "Fruit and Vegetable Consumption and Lung Cancer Risk: Updated Information from the European Prospective Investigation into Cancer and Nutrition (EPIC)." *Int J Cancer* 121(5) (Sep 1, 2007):1103–1114.

[382] Satia, J.A., A. Littman, C.G. Slatore, et al. "Long-Term Use of Beta-Carotene, Retinol, Lycopene, and Lutein Supplements and Lung Cancer Risk: Results from the VITamins And Lifestyle (VITAL) Study." *Am J Epidemiol* 169(7) (Apr 12009):815–828.

[383] Goralczyk, R. "Beta-Carotene and Lung Cancer in Smokers: Review of Hypotheses and Status of Research." *Nutr Cancer* 61(6) (2009):767–774.

[384] United States Department of Agriculture. "SR23 Page Reports." List of Nutrient Content in Foods http://www.ars.usda.gov/Services/docs.htm?docid=20957 . (accessed Aug 2011).

[385] Hoffer, A., A.W. Saul. *Orthomolecular Medicine for Everyone: Megavitamin Therapeu-*

tics for Families and Physicians. Laguna Beach CA: Basic Health Publications, 2008.

[386] Barakat, M.R., T.I. Metelitsina, J.C. DuPont, et al. "Effect of Niacin on Retinal Vascular Diameter in Patients with Age-Related Macular Degeneration." *Curr Eye Res.* 31(6-7) (Jul-Aug 2006):629–634. Millay, R.H., M.L. Klein, D.R. Illingworth. "Niacin Maculopathy." *Ophthalmology* 95(7) (1988):930–936. Dajani, H.M., A.K. Lauer "Optical Coherence Tomography Findings in Niacin Maculopathy." *Can J Ophthalmol* 41(2) (Apr 2006):197–200. L. Freisberg, T.J. Rolle, M.S. Ip, et al. "Diffuse Macular Edema in Niacin-Induced Maculopathy May Resolve With Dosage Decrease." *Retinal* Cases *Brief Rep* 5(3) (Sum 2011):227–228.

[387] Raczynska, K., B. Iwaszkiewicz-Bilikiewicz, W. Stozkowska, et al. "Clinical Evaluation of Provitamin B_5 Drops and Gel for Postoperative Treatment of Corneal and Conjuctival Injuries." *Klin Oczna* 105(3-4) (2003):175–178.

[388] Janoria, K.G., S. Hariharan, D. Paturi, et al. "Biotin Uptake by Rabbit Corneal Epithelial Cells: Role of Sodium-Dependent Multivitamin Transporter (SMVT)." *Curr Eye Res* 31(10) (Oct 2006):797–809.

[389] Mock. D.M. "Biotin" Chapter 28 in *Modern Nutrition in Health and Disease,* editors M.E.

Shils, J.A. Olson, M. Shike, et al., 9th ed. Baltimore, MD: Williams & Wilkins, 1999.

[390] Ames, B.N. "Low Micronutrient Intake May Accelerate the Degenerative Diseases of Aging through Allocation of Scarce Micronutrients by Triage." *Proc Natl Acad Sci USA.* 103 (2006):17589–17594.

[391] Elo, H.A., J. Korpela. "The Occurrence and Production of Avidin: A New Conception of the High-Affinity Biotin-Binding Protein." *Comp Biochem Physiol B* 78(1) (1984):15–20. M McGee, H. *On Food and Cooking: The Science and Lore of the Kitchen.* Rev. updated ed., New York, NY: Scribner; 2004.

[392] Christen, W.G., R.J. Glynn, E.Y. Chew, et al. "Folic Acid, Pyridoxine, and Cyanocobalamin Combination Treatment and Age-Related Macular Degeneration in Women: The Women's Antioxidant and Folic Acid Cardiovascular Study." *Arch Intern Med* 169(4) (Feb 23; 2009):335–341.

[393] Pacholok, S.M., J.J. Stuart. *Could It Be* B_{12}? *An Epidemic of Misdiagnoses.* 2nd ed. Fresno, CA: Linden Publishing, 2011.

[394] Linnér, E. "The Pressure Lowering Effect of Ascorbic Acid in Ocular Hypertension." *Acta Ophthalmol (Copenh)* 47(3) (1969):685–689, Boyd, H.H. "Eye Pressure Lowering Effect of Vitamin C." *J Orthomol Med* 10

(1995):165–168. Head, K.A. "Natural Therapies for Ocular Disorders, Part Two: Cataracts and Glaucoma." *Altern Med Rev* 6(2) (Apr 2001):141–166.

[395] Levy, T.E. *Curing the Incurable: Vitamin C, Infectious Diseases, and Toxins.* Henderson, NV: LivOn Books, 2002. Pfister, R.R., J.L. Haddox, D. Yuille-Barr. "The Combined Effect of Citrate/Ascorbate Treatment in Alkali-Injured Rabbit Eyes." *Cornea* 10(2) (Mai 1991):100–104.

[396] Pauling, L. *How to Live Longer And Feel Better.* Corvallis, OR: Oregon State University Press, 1986, 2006. Jacob, R.A. "Vitamin C." Chapter 29 in *Modern Nutrition in Health and Disease,* editors M.E. Shils, J.A. Olson, M. Shike, et al., 9th ed. Baltimore, MD: Williams & Wilkins, 1999. Hoffer, A., A.W. Saul. *Orthomolecular Medicine for Everyone: Megavitamin Therapeutics for Families and Physicians.* Laguna Beach, CA: Basic Health Publications, 2008. Hickey, S., A.W. Saul. *Vitamin C: The Real Story, the Remarkable and Controversial Healing Factor.* Laguna Beach, CA: Basic Health Publications, 2008.

[397] Montel-Hagen, A., M. Sitbon, N. Taylor. "Erythroid Glucose Transporters." *Curr Opin Hematol* 16(3) (May 2009):165–172. Spector, R "Nutrient Transport Systems in

Brain: 40 Years of Progress." *J Neurochem* 111(2) (Oct 2009):315–320.

[398] Hickey, S., A.W. Saul. *Vitamin C: The Real Story, the Remarkable and Controversial Healing Factor.* Laguna Beach, CA: Basic Health Publications, 2008.

[399] Frikke-Schmidt, H., P. Tveden-Nyborg, M.M. Birck, et al. "High Dietary Fat and Cholesterol Exacerbates Chronic Vitamin C Deficiency in Guinea Pigs." *Br J Nutr* 105(1) (Jan 2011):54–61.

[400] Levy, T.E. *Curing the Incurable: Vitamin C, Infectious Diseases, and Toxins.* Henderson, NV: LivOn Books, 2002.

[401] Dean, C. *The Magnesium Miracle.* New York, NY: Ballantine, 2007.

[402] Goodwin, J.S., M.R. Tangum. "Battling Quackery: Attitudes about Micronutrient Supplements in American Academic Medicine." *Arch Intern Med* 158(20) (Nov 9, 1998):2187–2191. Jacob, R.A. "Vitamin C." Chapter 29 in *Modern Nutrition in Health and Disease,* editors M. E Shils, J.A. Olson, M. Shike, et al., 9th ed. Baltimore, MD: Williams & Wilkins, 1999. Levy, T.E. *Curing the Incurable: Vitamin C, Infection: Diseases, and Toxins.* Henderson, NV: LivOn Books, 2002. Hickey, S., A.W. Saul. *Vitamin C: The Real Story, the Remarkable and Controversial Healing Factor.* Laguna Beach,

CA: Basic Health Publications, 2008. Robitaille, L., O.A. Mamer, W.H. Miller, et al. "Oxalic Acid Excretion after Intravenous Ascorbic Acid Administration." *Metabolism* 58(2) (Feb 2009):263–269.

[403] Hickey, S., A.W. Saul. *Vitamin C: The Real Story, the Remarkable and Controversial Healing Factor.* Laguna Beach, CA: Basic Health Publications, 2008.

[404] Levy, T.E. *Curing the Incurable: Vitamin C, Infectious Diseases, and Toxins.* Henderson, NV: LivOn Books, 2002.

[405] Jacob, R.A. "Vitamin C." Chapter 29 in *Modern Nutrition in Health and Disease,* editors M.E. Shils, J.A. Olson, M. Shike, et al., 9th ed Baltimore, MD: Williams & Wilkins, 1999.

[406] Hickey, S., A.W. Saul. *Vitamin C: The Real Story, the Remarkable and Controversial Healing Factor.* Laguna Beach, CA: Basic Health Publications, 2008.

[407] Council for Responsible Nutrition. "Fact Sheet: Are Vitamins and Minerals Safe for Persons with G6PD deficiency?" Washington, DC: Council for Responsible Nutrition, 2005. Available online at: http://www.crnusa.org/pdfs/CRN_G6PDDeficiency_0305.pdf. (accessed Aug 2011)

[408] Hickey, S., A.W. Saul. *Vitamin C: The Real Story, the Remarkable and Controversial*

Healing Factor. Laguna Beach, CA: Basic Health Publications, 2008. Padayatty, S.J., A.Y. Sun, Q. Chen, et al. "Vitamin C: Intravenous Use by Complementary and Alternative Medicine Practitioners and Adverse Effects." *PLoS One* 5(7) (Jul 7, 2010):e11414.

[409] Taylor, E.N., T.T. Fung, G.C. Curhan. "DASH-Style Diet Associates with Reduced Risk for Kidney Stones." *J Am Soc Nephrol* 20(10) (Oct 2009):2253–2259.

[410] Hickey, S., A.W. Saul. *Vitamin C: The Real Story, the Remarkable and Controversial Healing Factor.* Laguna Beach, CA: Basic Health Publications, 2008. Taylor, E.N., M.J. Stampfer, D.B. Mount, et al. "DASH-Style Diet and 24-Hour Urine Composition." *Clin J Am Soc Nephrol* 5(12) (Dec 2010):2315–2322.

[411] Hickey, S., A.W. Saul. *Vitamin C: The Real Story, the Remarkable and Controversial Healing Factor.* Laguna Beach, CA: Basic Health Publications, 2008.

[412] Oh, M.A., J. Uribarri. "Electrolytes, Water, and Acid-Base Balance." in *Modern Nutrition in Health and Disease,* editors M.E. Shils, J. A Olson, M. Shike, et al., 9th ed. Baltimore, MD: Williams & Wilkins, 1999.

[413] Hurrell, R., I. Egli. "Iron Bioavailability and Dietary Reference Values." *Am J Clin Nutr* 91(5) (May 2010):14615–14675.

[414] Conrad, M.E., J.N. Umbreit. "Iron Absorption and Transport-An Update." *Am J Hematol* 64(4) (Aug 2000):287–298

[415] Hickey, S., A.W. Saul. *Vitamin C: The Real Story, the Remarkable and Controversial Healing Factor.* Laguna Beach, CA: Basic Health Publications, 2008.

[416] Ibid.

[417] Holick, M.F. "Vitamin D: Extraskeletal Health." *Endocrinol Metab Clin North Am* 39(2) (Jun 2010):381–400. Holick, M.F. *The Vitamin D Solution: A 3-Step Strategy to Cure Our Most Common Health Problem.* New York, NY: Hudson Street Press, 2010.

[418] Parekh, N., R.J. Chappell, A.E. Millen, et al. "Association Between Vitamin D and Age-Related Macular Degeneration in the Third National Health and Nutrition Examination Survey, 1988 through 1994." *Arch Ophthalmol* 125(5) (May 2007):661–669. Mascitelli, L., F Pezzetta, M.R. Goldstein. "Macular Degeneration, Heart Disease, and Vitamin D." *Ophthalmology.* 117(1) (Jan 2010):194.

[419] Khalsa, S. *The Vitamin D Revolution: How the Power of This Amazing Vitamin Can Change Your Life.* Carlsbad, CA: Hay House, 2009.

[420] Jablonski, N.G., G. Chaplin. "Skin Deep." *Sci Am* 287(4) (Oct 2002):74–81.

[421] Jablonski, N.G., G. Chaplin. "Human Skin Pigmentation as an Adaptation to UV Radiation." *Proc Natl Acad Sci USA* 107(Suppl 2 (May 11, 2010):8962–8968.

[422] Ibid.

[423] Khalsa, S. *The Vitamin D Revolution: How the Power of This Amazing Vitamin Can Change Your Life.* Carlsbad, CA: Hay House, 2009 Holick, M.F. "Vitamin D: Extraskeletal Health." *Endocrinol Metab Clin North Am* 39(2) (Jun 2010):381–400. Holick, M.F. *The Vitamin D Solution: A 3-Step Strategy to Cure Our Most Common Health Problem.* New York, NY: Hudson Street Press, 2010.

[424] Institute of Medicine (IOM), Food and Nutrition Board. "Dietary Reference Intake for Calcium and Vitamin D." (Nov 30, 2010) Available online at: http://www.iom.edu/vitamind. (accessed Aug 2011)

[425] Holick, M.F. "The Vitamin D Defciency Pandemic and Consequences for Nonskeletal Health: Mechanisms of Action." *Mol Aspects Met* 29(6) (Dec 2008):361–368. Holick, M.F. "Vitamin D: Extraskeletal Health." *Endocrinol Metab Clin North Am* 39(2) (Jun 2010):381–40C Holick, M.F. *The Vitamin D Solution: A 3-Step Strategy to Cure Our Most Common Health Problem.* New York, NY: Hudson Street Press 2010.

[426] Heaney, R.P., M.F. Holick. "Why the IOM Recommendations for Vitamin D are Deficient." *J Bone Miner Res* 26(3) (Mar 24, 2011):455457.

[427] Holick, M.F. *The Vitamin D Solution: A 3-Step Strategy to Cure Our Most Common Health Problem.* New York, NY: Hudson Street Press, 2010.

[428] Khalsa, S. *The Vitamin D Revolution: How the Power of This Amazing Vitamin Can Change Your Life.* Carlsbad, CA: Hay House, 2009.

[429] Weaver, C.M., R.P. Heaney "Calcium." Chapter 7 in *Modern Nutrition in Health and Disease,* editors M.E. Shils, J.A. Olson, M. Shik, et al., 9th ed. Baltimore, MD: Williams & Wilkins, 1999.

[430] Dean, C. *The Magnesium Miracle.* New York, NY: Ballantine, 2007.

[431] Shils, M.E. "Magnesium." Chapter 9 in *Modern Nutrition in Health and Disease,* editors M.E. Shils, J.A. Olson, M. Shike, et al., 9th ed. Baltimore, MD: Williams & Wilkins, 1999.

[432] Ibid.

[433] Li, F.Y., B. Chaigne-Delalande, C. Kanellopoulou, et al. "Second Messenger Role for Mg2+ Revealed by Human T-Cell Immunodeficiency." *Nature* 475(7357) (Jul 27, 2011):471–476.

[434] Dean, C. *The Magnesium Miracle.* New York, NY: Ballantine, 2007.

[435] Hoffer, A., A.W. Saul. *Orthomolecular Medicine for Everyone: Megavitamin Therapeutics for Families and Physicians.* Laguna Beach, CA: Basic Health Publications, 2008.

[436] Ames, B.N. "Low Micronutrient Intake May Accelerate the Degenerative Diseases of Aging through Allocation of Scarce Micronutrients by Triage." *Proc Natl Acad Sci USA.* 103 (2006):17589–17594. Dean, C. *The Magnesium Miracle.* New York, NY: Ballantine, 2007.

[437] Dean, C. *The Magnesium Miracle.* New York, NY: Ballantine, 2007.

[438] Ibid.

[439] Ibid.

[440] Shils, M.E. "Magnesium." Chapter 9 in *Modern Nutrition in Health and Disease,* editors M.E. Shils, J.A. Olson, M. Shike, et al., 9th ed Baltimore, MD: Williams & Wilkins, 1999.

[441] United States Department of Agriculture. "SR23Page Reports." List of Nutrient Content in Foods. http://www.ars.usda.gov/Services/docs.htm?docid=20957 . (accessed Aug 2011).

[442] Dean, C. *The Magnesium Miracle.* New York, NY: Ballantine, 2007.

[443] Hoffer, A., A.W. Saul. *Orthomolecular Medicine for Everyone: Megavitamin Therapeu-*

tics for Families and Physicians. Laguna Beach CA: Basic Health Publications, 2008.

[444] Mehta, J., D. LI, J.L. Mehta. "Vitamins C and E Prolong Time to Arterial Thrombosis in Rats." *J Nutr* 129(1) (Jan 1999):109–112 Traber, M.G.. "Does Vitamin E Decrease Heart Attack Risk? Summary and Implications with Respect to Dietary Recommendations." *J Nutr* 131 (2001):3955–3975.

[445] Schürks, M., R.J. Glynn, P.M. Rist, et al. "Effects of Vitamin E on Stroke Subtypes: Meta-Analysis of Randomised Controlled Trials." *BMJ.* 341 (Nov 4, 2010):c57–02.

[446] Levy, T.E. *Stop America's #1 Killer: Reversible Vitamin Deficiency Found to be Origin of All Coronary Heart Disease.* Henderson, NV LivOn Books, 2006.

[447] Miller, E.R. III, R. Pastor-Barriuso, D. Dalal, et al. "Meta-Analysis: High-Dosage Vitamin E Supplementation May Increase All-Cause Mortality." *Ann Intern Med* 142(1) (Jan 4, 2005):37–46.

[448] Yusuf, S., G. Dagenais, J. Pogue, et al. "Vitamin E Supplementation and Cardiovascular Events in High-Risk Patients: The Heart Outcomes Prevention Evaluation Study Investigators." *N Engl J Med* 342(3) (Jan 20, 2000):154–160.

[449] Schürks, M., R.J. Glynn, P.M. Rist, et al. "Effects of Vitamin E on Stroke Subtypes: Meta-

Analysis of Randomised Controlled Trials." *BMJ.* 341 (Nov 4, 2010):c5702.

[450] Kurl, S., T.P. Tuomainen, J.A. Laukkanen, et al. "Plasma Vitamin C Modifies the Association between Hypertension and Risk of Stroke." *Stroke* 33(6) (Jun 2002):1568–1573.

[451] Shargorodsky, M., O. Debby, Z. Matas, et al. "Effect of Long-Term Treatment with Antioxidants (Vitamin C, Vitamin E, Coenzyme Q_{10} and Selenium) on Arterial Compliance, Humoral Factors and Inflammatory Markers in Patients with Multiple Cardiovascular Risk Factors." *Nutr Metab (Lond)* 7 (Jul 6, 2010):55.

[452] Brigelius-Flohe, R., F. Galli. "Vitamin E: A Vitamin Still Awaiting the Detection of Its Biological Function." *Mol. Nutr Food Res* 54(5 (May 2010):583–587.

[453] Azzi, A. "Molecular Mechanism of Alpha-Tocopherol Action." *Free Radic Biol Med* 43(1) (Jul 1, 2007):16–21.

[454] Jensen, S.K., C. Lauridsen. "Alpha-Tocopherol Stereo isomers." *Vitam Horm* 76 (2007):281–308.

[455] Papas, A. *The Vitamin E Factor: The Miraculous Antioxidant for the Prevention and Treatment of Heart disease, Cancer, and Aging.* New York, NY: HarperCollins, 1999. Sen, C.K., S. Khanna, S. Roy. "Tocotrienols: Vitamin E Beyond Tocopherols." *Life Sci* 78(18)

(Mar 27,2006):2088–2098. Jensen, S.K., C. Lauridsen. "Alpha-Tocopherol Stereoisomers." *Vitam Horm* 76 (2007):281–308. Colombo, M.L. "An Update on Vitamin E, Tocopherol and Tocotrienol-Perspectives." *Molecules* 15(4) (Mar 24, 2010):2103–2113

[456] Azzi, A. "Molecular Mechanism of Alpha-Tocopherol Action." *Free Radic Biol Med* 43(1) (Jul 1, 2007):16–21. Banks, R., J.R. Speakman, C. Selman. "Vitamin E Supplementation and Mammalian Lifespan." *Mol Nutr Food Res* 54(5) (May 2010):719–725.

[457] Tanito, M., N. Itoh, Y. Yoshida, et al. "Distribution of Tocopherols and Tocotrienols to Rat Ocular Tissues after Topical Ophthalmic Administration." *Lipids* 39(5) (May 2004):469–474.

[458] Sen, C.K., S. Khanna, S. Roy. "Tocotrienols: Vitamin E Beyond Tocopherols." *Life Sci* 78(18) (Mar 27,2006):2088–2098.

[459] Berson, E.L., B. Rosner, M.A. Sandberg, et al. "A Randomized Trial of Vitamin A and Vitamin E Supplementation for Retinitis Pigmentosa." *Arch Ophthalmol* 111(6) (Jun 1993):761–772.

Christen, W.G., R.J. Glynn, E.Y. Chew, et al. "Vitamin E and Age-Related Macular Degeneration in a Randomized Trial of Women." *Ophthalmology* 117(6) (Jun 2010):1163–1168. Christen, W.G., R.J. Glynn, H.D. Sesso, et al. "Age-Related

Cataract in a Randomized Trial of Vitamins E and C in Men." *Arch Ophthalmol* 128(11) (Nov 2010):1397–1405.

[460] Papas, A. *The Vitamin E Factor: The Miraculous Antioxidant for the Prevention and Treatment of Heart disease, Cancer, and Aging.* New York, NY: HarperCollins, 1999. Jensen, S.K., C. Lauridsen. "Alpha-Tocopherol Stereo isomers." *Vitam Horm* 76 (2007):281–308.

[461] Banks, R., J.R. Speakman, C. Selman. "Vitamin E Supplementation and Mammalian Lifespan." *Mol Nutr Food Res* 54(5) (Ma) 2010):719–725.

[462] Berson, E.L., B. Rosner, M.A. Sandberg, et al. "A Randomized Trial of Vitamin A and Vitamin E Supplementation for Retinitis Pigmentosa." *Arch Ophthalmol* 111(6) (Jun 1993):761–772. Christen, W.G., R.J. Glynn, E.Y. Chew, et al. "Vitamin E and Age-Related Macular Degeneration in a Randomized Trial of Women." *Ophthalmology* 117(6) (Jun 2010):1163–1168. Christen, W.G., R.J. Glynn, H.D. Sesso, et al. "Age-Related Cataract in a Randomized Trial of Vitamins E and C in Men." *Arch Ophthalmol* 128(11) (Nov 2010):1397–1405.

[463] Jacob, R.A. "Vitamin C." Chapter 29 in *Modern Nutrition in Health and Disease,* editors M.E. Shils, J.A. Olson, M. Shike, et al.,

9th ed Baltimore, MD: Williams & Wilkins, 1999.

[464] Hoffer, A., A.W. Saul. *Orthomolecular Medicine for Everyone: Megavitamin Therapeutics for Families and Physicians.* Laguna Beach CA: Basic Health Publications, 2008.

[465] Banks, R., J.R. Speakman, C. Selman. "Vitamin E Supplementation and Mammalian Lifespan." *Mol Nutr Food Res* 54(5) (Ma, 2010):719–725.

[466] Traber, M.G. "Regulation of Xenobiotic Metabolism, the Only Signaling Function of Alpha-Tocopherol?" *Mol Nutr Food Res* 54(5 (May 2010):661–668.

[467] Kurl, S., T.P. Tuomainen, J.A. Laukkanen, et al. "Plasma Vitamin C Modifies the Association between Hypertension and Risk of Stroke." *Stroke* 33(6) (Jun 2002):1568–1573. Levy, T.E. *Stop America's #1 Killer: Reversible Vitamin Deficiency Found to be Origin of All Coronary Heart Disease.* Henderson, NV: LivOn Books, 2006. Shargorodsky, M., O. Debby, Z. Matas, et al. "Effect of Long-Term Treatment with Antioxidants (Vitamin C, Vitamin E, Coenzyme Q_{10} and Selenium) on Arterial Compliance, Humoral Factors and Inflammatory Markers in Patients with Multiple Cardiovascular Risk Factors." *Nutr Metab (Lond)* 7 (Jul 6, 2010):55. Pfister, R., S.J. Sharp, R. Luben, et al. "Plasma Vitamin C Predicts Inci-

dent Heart Failure in Men and Women in European Prospective Investigation into Cancer and Nutrition Norfolk Prospective Study." *Am Heart J* 162(2) (Aug 2011):246–253.

[468] McCann, J.C., B.N. Ames. "Vitamin K, An Example of Triage Theory: Is Micronutrient Inadequacy Linked to Diseases of Aging?" *Am Clin Nutr* 90 (Oct 2009):889–907.

[469] Borràs, T., N. Comes. "Evidence for a Calcification Process in the Trabecular Meshwork." *Exp Eye Res.* 88(4) (Apr 2009):738–746. 470. Ibid.

[471] Carrié, I., G. Ferland, M.S. Obin. "Effects of Long-Term Vitamin K (Phylloquinone) Intake on Retina Aging." *Nutr Neurosci* 6(6) (Dec 2003):351–359.

[472] Emery, T.F. *Iron and your Health: Facts and Fallacies.* Boca Raton, FL: CRC Press, 1991. Fairbanks, V.F. "Iron in Medicine and Nutrition." Chapter 10 in *Modern Nutrition in Health and Disease,* editors M.E. Shils, J.A. Olson, M. Shike, et al., 9th ed. Baltimore, MI Williams & Wilkins, 1999.

[473] Emery, T.F. *Iron and your Health: Facts and Fallacies.* Boca Raton, FL: CRC Press, 1991. Hurrell, R., I. Egli. "Iron Bioavailability an Dietary Reference Values." *Am J Clin Nutr* 91(5) (May 2010):1461S-14675.

[474] Killilea, D.W., S.L. Wong, H.S. Cahaya, et al. "Iron Accumulation during Cellular Senes-

cence." *Annals NY Acad Sci* 1019 (Jun 2004):365–367

[475] Richer, S., W. Stiles, C. Thomas. "Molecular Medicine in Ophthalmic Care." *Optometry* 80(12) (Dec 2009):695–701.

[476] Terman, A., U.T. Brunk. "Oxidative Stress, Accumulation of Biological Garbage and Aging." *Antioxid Redox Signal* 8(1–2) (Jan-Feb 2006):197–204.

[477] Knutson, M.D., P.B. Walter, B.N. Ames, et al. "Both Iron Deficiency and Daily Iron Supplements Increase Lipid Peroxidation in Rats." *J Nutr*130(2000):621–628.

[478] Emery, *T.F. Iron and your Health: Facts and Fallacies.* Boca Raton, FL: CRC Press, 1991.

[479] Conrad, M.E., J.N. Umbreit "Iron Absorption and Transport-An Update." *Am J Hcmatol* 64(4) (Aug 2000):287–298.

[480] Ibid.

[481] Emery, T.F. *Iron and your Health: Facts and Fallacies.* Boca Raton, FL: CRC Press, 1991. Hoffer, A., A.W. Saul. *Orthomoleculai Medicine for Everyone: Megavitamin Therapeutics for Families and Physicians.* Laguna Beach, CA: Basic Health Publications, 2008.

[482] Hoffer, A., A.W. Saul. *Orthomolecular Medicine for Everyone: Megavitamin Therapeutics for Families and Physicians.* Laguna Beach CA: Basic Health Publications, 2008.

Saper, R.B., R. Rash. "Zinc: An Essential Micronutrient." *Am Fam Physician* 79(9) (May 1, 2009):768772. Little, P.J., R. Bhattacharya, A.E. Moreyra, et al. "Zinc and Cardiovascular Disease." *Nutrition* 26(11-12) (Nov-Dec 2010):1050–1057.

[483] Head, K.A. "Natural Therapies for Ocular Disorders, Part One: Diseases of the Retina." *Altern Med Rev* 4(5) (Oct 1999):342–359.

[484] King, J.C., C.L. Keen. "Zinc" Chapter 11 in *Modern Nutrition in Health and Disease,* editors M.E. Shils, J.A. Olson, M. Shike, et al., 9th ed. Baltimore, MD: Williams & Wilkins, 1999.

[485] Saper, R.B., R. Rash. "Zinc: An Essential Micro nutrient." *Am Fam Physician* 79(9) (May 1, 2009):768–772.

[486] King, J.C., C.L. Keen. "Zinc." Chapter 11 in *Modern Nutrition in Health and Disease,* editors M.E. Shils, J.A. Olson, M. Shike, et al., 9t1 ed. Baltimore, MD: Williams & Wilkins, 1999. Turnlund, J.R. "Copper." Chapter 12 King, J.C., C.L. Keen. "Zinc." Chapter 11 in *Modern Nutrition in Health and Disease,* editors M.E. Shils, J.A. Olson, M. Shike, et al., 9th ed. Baltimore, MD: Williams & Wilkins, 1999. Hoffer, A.A.W. Saul. *Orthomolecular Medicine for Everyone: Megavitamin Therapeutics for Families and*

Physicians. Laguna Beach, CA: Basic Health Publications, 2008.

[487] Maggini, S., E.S. Wintergerst, S. Beveridge, et al. "Selected Vitamins and Trace Elements Support Immune Function by Strengthening Epithelial Barriers and Cellular and Humoral Immune Responses." *Br J Nutr* 98 Suppl 1 (Oct 2007):529–35.

[488] Burk, R.F., O.A. Levander "Selenium." Chapter 14 in *Modern Nutrition in Health and Disease,* editors M.E. Shils, J.A. Olson, M. Shike, et al., 9th ed. Baltimore, MD: Williams & Wilkins, 1999.

[489] Ibid.

[490] Hoffer, A., A.W. Saul. *Orthomolecular Medicine for Everyone: Megavitamin Therapeutics for Families and Physicians.* Laguna Beach, CA: Basic Health Publications, 2008.

[491] Burk, R.F., O.A. Levander "Selenium." Chapter 14 in *Modern Nutrition in Health and Disease,* editors M.E. Shils, J.A. Olson, M. Shike, et al., 9th ed. Baltimore, MD: Williams & Wilkins, 1999. Waters, D.J., S. Shen, L.T. Glickman, et al. "Prostate Cancer Risk and DN7 Damage: Translational Significance of Selenium Supplementation in a Canine Model." *Carcinogenesis* 26(7) (Jul 2005):1256–1262.

[492] United States Department of Agriculture. "SR23Page Reports." List of Nutrient Content

in Foods http://www.ars.usda.gov/Services/docs.htm?docid=20957 (accessed Aug 2011).

[493] Waters, D.J., S. Shen, L.T. Glickman, et al. "Prostate Cancer Risk and DNA Damage: Translational Significance of Seleniun Supplementation in a Canine Model." *Carcinogenesis* 26(7) (Jul 2005):1256–1262.

[494] Head, K.A. "Natural Therapies for Ocular Disorders, Part One: Diseases of the Retina." *Altern Med Rev* 4(5) (Oct 1999):342–359.

[495] Nielsen, F.H. "Ultratrace Minerals." Chapter 16 in *Modern Nutrition in Health and Disease,* editors M.E. Shils, J.A. Olson, M. Shike, al., 9th ed. Baltimore, MD: Williams & Wilkins, 1999.

[496] Organisciak, D.T., D.K. Vaughan. "Retinal Light Damage: Mechanisms and Protection." *Prog Retin Eye Res* 29(2) (Mar 2010):113–134.

[497] Ibid.

[498] Vanderhaeghe, L.R., K. Karst. *Healthy Fats for Life: Preventing and Treating Common Health Problems with Essential Fatty Acids. 2nd* ed. Toronto, ON: John Wiley and Sons Canada, 2004.

[499] Simopoulos, A.P., J. Robinson. *The Omega Diet: The Lifesaving Nutritional Program Based on the Diet of the Island of Crete.* New York NY: HarperCollins, 1999. Saul, A. *Doctor Yourself. Natural Healing That Works.* Laguna

Beach, CA: Basic Health Publications, 2003. Pollan, *M. In Defense of Food: An Eater's Manifesto.* New York, NY: Penguin, 2009. Hoffer, A., A.W. Saul. *Orthomolecular Medicine for Everyone: Megavitamin Therapeutics for Families and Physicians.* Laguna Beach, CA: Basic Health Publications, 2008.

[500] Wong, I.Y., S.C. Koo, C.W. Chan. "Prevention of Age-Related Macular Degeneration." *Int Ophthalmol* 31(1) (Feb 2011):73–82.

[501] Lien, E.L., B.R. Hammond. "Nutritional Influences on Visual Development and Function." *Prog Retin Eye Res* 30(3) (May 2011):188203.

[502] Ibid.

[503] Rhone, M., A. Basu. "Phytochemicals and Age-Related Eye Diseases." *Nutr Rev* 66(8) (Aug 2008):465–472.

[504] Berson, E.L., B. Rosner, M.A. Sandberg, et al. "Clinical Trial of Lutein in Patients with Retinitis Pigmentosa Receiving Vitamin A." *Arch Ophthalmol* 128(4) (Apr 2010):403–411.

[505] Wong, I.Y., S.C. Koo, C.W. Chan. "Prevention of Age-Related Macular Degeneration." *Int Ophthalmol* 31(1) (Feb 2011):73–82. 506. Ibid.

[507] Pashkow, F.J., D.G. Watumull, C.L. Campbell. "Astaxanthin: a Novel Potential Treatment for Oxidative Stress and Inflammation in Cardiovascular Disease." *Am J Cardiol* 101(10A) (May 22, 2008):58D-68D.

[508] Osborne, N.N. "Pathogenesis of Ganglion "Cell Death" in Glaucoma and Neuroprotection: Focus on Ganglion Cell Axonal Mitochondria." *Prog Brain Res* 173 (2008):339–352.

[509] Packer, L. "Antioxidant Properties of Lipoic Aid and Its Therapeutic Effects in Prevention of Diabetes Complications and Cataracts." *Ann NY Acad Sci* 738 (Nov 17, 1994):257–264.

[510] Mijnhout, G.S., A. Alkhalaf, N. Kleefstra, et al. "Alpha Lipoic Acid: A New Treatment for Neuropathic Pain in Patients with Diabetes?" *Neth J Med* 68(4) (Apr 2010):158–162.

[511] Janoria, K.G., S. Hariharan, D. Paturi, et al. "Biotin Uptake by Rabbit Corneal Epithelial Cells: Role of Sodium-Dependen Multivitamin Transporter (SMVT)." *Curr Eye Res* 31(10) (Oct 2006):797–809.

[512] Packer, L. "Antioxidant Properties of Lipoic Aid and Its Therapeutic Effects in Prevention of Diabetes Complications and Cataracts." *Ann NY Acad Sci* 738 (Nov 17, 1994):257–264.

[513] Stoyanovsky, D.A., R. Goldman, R.M. Darrow, et al. "Endogenous Ascorbate Regenerates Vitamin E in the Retina Directly and in Combination with Exogenous Dihydrolipoic Acid." *Curr Eye Res* 14(3) (Mar 1995):181–189. Head, K.A. "Natural Therapies for Ocular Disorders, Part Two: Cataracts and Glaucoma." *Altern Med Rev* 6(2) (Apr 2001):141–166. Komeima, K., B.S. Rogers, L. Lu, et at "An-

tioxidants Reduce Cone Cell Death in a Model of Retinitis Pigmentosa." *Proc Natl Acad Sci USA* 103(30) (Jul 25, 2006):11300–11305 Komeima, K., B.S. Rogers, P.A. Campochiaro. "Antioxidants Slow Photoreceptor Cell Death in Mouse Models of Retinitis Pigmentosa." *J Cell Physiol* 213(3) (Dec 2007):809–815.

[514] Head, K.A. "Natural Therapies for Ocular Disorders, Part Two: Cataracts and Glaucoma." *Altern Med Rev* 6(2) (Apr 2001):141–166.

[515] Packer, L. "Antioxidant Properties of Lipoic Aid and Its Therapeutic Effects in Prevention of Diabetes Complications and Cataracts." *Ann NY Acad Sci* 738 (Nov 17, 1994):257–264.

[516] Hoffer, A., A.W. Saul. *Orthomolecular Medicine for Everyone: Megavitamin Therapeutics for Families and Physicians.* Laguna Bead CA: Basic Health Publications, 2008.

[517] Cagini, C., A. Leontiadis, M.A. Ricci, et al. "Study of Alpha-Lipoic Acid penetration in the Human Aqueous after Topical Administration." *Clin Experiment Ophthalmol* 38(6) (Aug 2010):572–576.

[518] Taylor, F.R. "Nutraceuticals and Headache: The Biological Basis." *Headache* 51(3) (Mar 2011):484–501.

[519] Qu, J., Y. Kaufman, I. Washington. "Coenzyme Q_{10} in the Human Retina." *Invest Ophthalmol Vis Sci* 50(4) (Apr 2009):1814–1818.

[520] Hathcock, J.N., A. Shao. "Risk Assessment for Coenzyme Q_{10} (Ubiquinone)." *Regul Toxicol Pharmacol* 45(3) (Aug 2006):282–28! Hyson, H.C., K. Kieburtz, I. Shoulson, et al. "Safety and Tolerability of High-Dosage Coenzyme Q_{10} in Huntington's Disease and Healthy Subjects." *Mov Disord* 25(12) (Sep 15, 2010):1924–1928.

[521] Hickey, S., A.W. Saul. *Vitamin C: The Real Story, the Remarkable and Controversial Healing Factor.* Laguna Beach, CA: Basic Health Publications, 2008. Hoffer, A., A.W. Saul. *Orthomolecular Medicine for Everyone: Megavitamin Therapeutics for Families and Physicians.* Laguna Beach, CA: Basic Health Publications, 2008.

[522] Akyol-Salman, I., S. Azizi, U. Mumcu, et al. "Efficacy of Topical N-Acetylcysteine in the Treatment of Meibomian Gland Dysfunction." *Ocul Pharmacol Ther* 26(4) (Aug 2010):329–333.

[523] Urgancioglu, B., K. Bilgihan, D. Engin, et al. "Topical N-Acetylcysteine Reduces Interleukin-1-Alpha in Tear Fluid After Laser Subepithelial Keratectomy." *Eur J Ophthalmol* 19(4) (Jul-Aug 2009):554–559.

[524] Gerona, G., D. Lopez, M. Palmero, et al. "Antioxidant N-Acetyl-Cysteine Protects Retinal Pigmented Epithelial Cells from Long-Term

Hypoxia Changes in Gene Expression." *J Ocul Pharmacol Ther* 26(4) (Aug 2010):309–314.
[525] Lei, H., G. Velez, J. Cui, et al. "N-Acetylcysteine Suppresses Retinal Detachment in an Experimental Model of Proliferative Vitreoretinopathy." *Am J Pathol* 177(1) (Jul 2010):132–140.
[526] Fletcher, A.E. "Controversy over "Contradiction": Should Randomized Trials Always Trump Observational Studies?" *Am J Ophthalmol* 147(3) (Mar 2009):384–386.
[527] Qu, J., Y. Kaufman, I. Washington. "Coenzyme Q_{10} in the Human Retina." *Invest Ophthalmol Vis Sci* 50(4) (Apr 2009):1814–1818. 528 Bartlett, H., F. Eperjesi. "An Ideal Ocular Nutritional Supplement?" *Ophthalmic Physiol Opt* 24(4) (Jul 2004):339–349.
[529] Stoyanovsky, D.A., R. Goldman, R.M. Darrow, et al. "Endogenous Ascorbate Regenerates Vitamin E in the Retina Directly and in Combination with Exogenous Dihydrolipoic Acid." *Curr Eye Res* 14(3) (Mar 1995):181–189. Jacob, R.A. "Vitamin C." Chapter 29 in *Modern Nutrition in Health and Disease,* editors M.E. Shils, J.A. Olson, M. Shike, et al., 9th ed. Baltimore, MD: Williams & Wilkins, 1999 Hickey, S., A.W. Saul. *Vitamin C: The Real Story, the Remarkable and Controversial Healing Factor.* Lagu-

na Beach, CA: Basic Health Publications, 2008.

[530] Mendiratta, S., Z.C. Qu, J.M. May. "Erythrocyte Ascorbate Recycling: Antioxidant Effects in Blood." *Free Radic Biol Med* 24(5) (Mal 15,1998):789–797.

[531] Stoyanovsky, D.A., R. Goldman, R.M. Darrow, et al. "Endogenous Ascorbate Regenerates Vitamin E in the Retina Directly and in Combination with Exogenous Dihydrolipoic Acid." *Curr Eye Res* 14(3) (Mar 1995):181–189.

[532] Head, K.A. "Natural Therapies for Ocular Disorders, Part One: Diseases of the Retina." *Altern Med Rev* 4(5) (Oct 1999):342–359. Head K.A. "Natural Therapies for Ocular Disorders, Part Two: Cataracts and Glaucoma." *Altern Med Rev* 6(2) (Apr 2001):141–166. Gaby, A. R "Nutritional Therapies for Ocular Disorders: Part Three." *Altern Med Rev* 13(3) (Sep 2008):191–204. Johnson, E.J. "Age-Related Macular Degeneration and Antioxidant Vitamins: Recent Findings." *Curr Opin Clin Nutr Metab Care* 13(1) (Jan 2010):28–33

[533] Williams, R.J., D.K. Kalita. A *Physician's Handbook on Orthomolecular Medicine.* Chicago, IL: Keats Pub, 1979. Pauling, L. *How to Live Longer And Feel Better.* Corvallis, OR: Oregon State University Press, 1986,

2006. Saul, A. *Doctor Yourself Natural Healing That Works.* Laguna Beach, CA: Basic Health Publications, 2003. Ames, B.N. "Low Micronutrient Intake May Accelerate the Degenerative Diseases of Aging through Allocation of Scarce Micronutrients by Triage." *Proc Natl Acad Sci USA.* 103 (2006):17589–17594. Ames, B.N. "Optima Micronutrients Delay Mitochondrial Decay and Age-associated Diseases." *Mech Ageing Dev* 131 (2010):473–479. Hickey, S., A.W. Saul. *Vitamin C: The Real Story, the Remarkable and Controversial Healing Factor.* Laguna Beach, CA: Basic Health Publications, 2008. Hoffer, A A.W. Saul. *Orthomolecular Medicine for Everyone: Megavitamin Therapeutics for Families and Physicians.* Laguna Beach, CA: Basic Health Publications, 2008.

[534] Hoffer, A., A.W. Saul. *Orthomolecular Medicine for Everyone: Megavitamin Therapeutics for Families and Physicians.* Laguna Bead CA: Basic Health Publications, 2008.

[535] Pauling, L. *How to Live Longer And Feel Better.* Corvallis, OR: Oregon State University Press, 1986, 2006. Hoffer, A., A.W. Saul. *Orthomolecular Medicine for Everyone: Megavitamin Therapeutics for Families and Physicians.* Laguna Beach, CA: Basic Health Publications, 2008.

[536] Williams, R.J., G. Deason. "Individuality in Vitamin C Needs." *Proc Natl Acad Sci USA* 57(6) (Jun 1967):1638–1641. Packer, I "Protective Role of Vitamin E in Biological Systems." *Am J Clin Nutr* 53 (1991):10505–10555. Hickey, S., A.W. Saul. *Vitamin C: The Read Story, the Remarkable and Controversial Healing Factor.* Laguna Beach, CA: Basic Health Publications, 2008.

[537] Pauling, L. *How to Live Longer And Feel Better.* Corvallis, OR: Oregon State University Press, 1986, 2006. Hickey, S., A.W. Saul. *Vitamin C: The Real Story, the Remarkable and Controversial Healing Factor.* Laguna Beach, CA: Basic Health Publications, 2008.

[538] Hickey, S., A.W. Saul. *Vitamin C: The Real Story, the Remarkable and Controversial Healing Factor.* Laguna Beach, CA: Basic Health Publications, 2008.

[539] Papas, A. *The Vitamin E Factor: The Miraculous Antioxidant for the Prevention and Treatment of Heart disease, Cancer, and Aging.* New York, NY: HarperCollins, 1999. Hoffer, A., A.W. Saul. *Orthomolecular Medicine for Everyone: Megavitamin Therapeutics for Families an Physicians.* Laguna Beach, CA: Basic Health Publications, 2008.

[540] Head, K.A. "Natural Therapies for Ocular Disorders, Part One: Diseases of the Retina." *Altern Med Rev* 4(5) (Oct 1999):342–359. Head, K.A. "Natural Therapies for Ocular Disorders, Part Two: Cataracts and Glaucoma." *Altern Med Rev* 6(2) (Apr 2001):141–166.

ABOUT THE AUTHOR

Robert Smith is a research scientist, focusing on the function of retinal circuitry. He received his Ph.D. and did his postdoctoral fellowship at the University of Pennsylvania, where he was appointed as a research-track scientist. He has continued to work on the circuitry of the retina at the University of Pennsylvania for the last two decades. Dr. Smith's research focuses on the how and why of neural circuits. He studies the signal-processing function of retinal neurons and the circuits they form. He is an expert in the physiology and biophysical properties of neurons and in constructing realistic biophysical computational models of neural circuits of the retina. Dr. Smith has studied many aspects of retinal circuitry, including color coding, singlephoton detection at night, contrast coding, motion processing, and a variety of electrical and chemical signaling circuits in the retina. He has written many research articles published in scientific journals, has served on review panels for grant applications to the National Institutes for Health, and is a regular attendee at international retina and vision conferences. He is an avid photographer of nature and landscapes.

Robert Smith's interest in vision started as a child, from a passionate interest in nature and photography. He taught himself analog and digital electronics as a young adult. He then built a homemade microcomputer and proceeded to learn software. For several years he worked at the University of Pennsylvania as an engineer designing data acquisition hardware and software for neuroscientists. He then worked for several years as a software engineer in the Department of Neuroscience at the University, where he designed graphics software for the serial reconstruction of neural circuits from electron microscope images and became familiar with neural circuits and their function. He went on to graduate school in Neuroscience at the University and wrote his thesis on computational modeling of the photoreceptor-horizontal cell network. Dr. Smith continues to work on this layer of the retina. His work in the circuitry of the retina is unique, utilizing the principles of electronics, software programming, and neuroscience to learn how the retina can see and categorize the visual world. This work is fundamental for understanding how the eye sees, and has helped clinical researchers to better understand the basis of eye disease.

Printed in Dunstable, United Kingdom

91336856R00197